KU-215-275

EXERCISE
BALL FOR
WEIGHT
LOSS

EXERCISE BALL FOR WEIGHT LOSS

LUCY KNIGHT

KYLE CATHIE LIMITED

First published in Great Britain in 2005 by
Kyle Cathie Limited,122 Arlington Road,
London NW1 7HP
general.enquiries@kyle-cathie.com
www.kyle-cathie.com

10 9 8 7 6 5 4 3

ISBN 978 1 85626 613 0

All rights reserved. No reproduction, copy or
transmission of this publication may be made
without written permission. No paragraph of
this publication may be reproduced, copied
or transmitted save with written permission
or in accordance with the provision of the
Copyright Act 1956 (as amended). Any person
who does any unauthorised act in relation to
this publication may be liable to criminal
prosecution and civil claims for damages.

Text © 2005 Lucy Knight
Photography © 2005 Glenn Burnip
Additional photography: Francesca Yorke
(pages 5, 118-133, 136-138 and (r)141)

Project editor: Sarah Epton
Copy editor: Anne Newman
Editorial assistant: Vicki Murrell
Food stylist: Liz Collins
Designer: Becky Willis
Production: Sha Huxtable and Alice Holloway

Lucy Knight is hereby identified as the author
of this work in accordance with Section 77 of
the Copyright, Designs and Patents Act 1988.

A CIP catalogue record for this book is
available from the British Library.

Colour separations by Scanhouse, Malaysia
Printed and bound in Singapore by KHL

Author's Acknowledgements
To my darling Ken for your constant support,
love, coaching and unending belief in me.
What you have given me is immeasurable –
thank you so very much.

And to the rest of my family, especially Mum,
Dad, Jo and little Jess for being the solid
people in my life, and thanks Mum for
supplying some delicious recipes for this book.

Thanks also to the people I have learnt from
along the way, teachers, colleagues and
friends: you have all contributed indirectly
to this book.

Thanks must also go to my publisher Kyle
Cathie, editor Sarah Epton, photographers
Glenn Burnip and Francesca Yorke, food
stylist Liz Collins and designer Becky Willis.

Thanks also to USA Pro for supplying the
clothing.

Note:
The author and publisher cannot accept
any responsibility for misadventure resulting
from the practice of any of the techniques or
principles in this book. It is not intended to be
and should not be used as guidance for the
treatment of serious health problems; please
refer to a medical professional if you have
concerns about any aspect of your condition
or fitness level.

CONTENTS

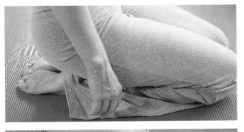
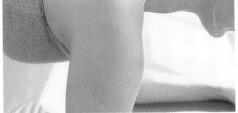
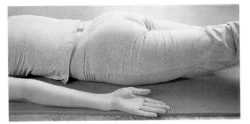
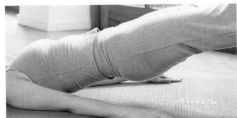
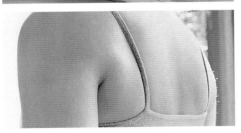
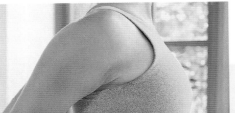

INTRODUCTION

Exercise Ball for Weight Loss is a unique book in which you will discover the many amazing qualities of the ball – you will learn how to isolate, stretch and strengthen every muscle group in your body, as well as how to prevent back pain and postural problems. This, coupled with a sensible approach to healthy eating, will bring about some staggering, long-lasting changes in your body shape. Not only will you benefit from fantastic results, you will also find a determination within yourself that you never knew existed. And you will soon realise how much fun exercise can and should be as you roll around on your oversized vinyl ball. I promise you won't be able to do this without laughing. And falling off is inevitable!

The aim

Although weight loss is the ultimate aim of the book – hence the title – you should not allow yourself to get too hung up on worrying about what the scales say. Instead, channel your energy into changing your eating habits for the better: feed your body with foods that are beneficial, that enhance your mood, aid the smooth functioning of your body's systems, and do not make you feel bloated or sluggish.

This book will set you on your way to making life-long changes. The workouts, together with some delicious recipe ideas and an eating plan will get you started, but in time I want you to use and adapt the information to create a balanced diet and exercise programme of your own – one that really works for you. I'm just here to motivate and give you a kick-start!

Once all these changes are in place, your body will naturally alter its shape and weight. In fact, in keeping with my no-scales policy, I am going to recommend an amazingly primitive, non-technical way of monitoring your progress: the good old tape measure. If you don't already have one, it should cost you no more than the price of

a cup of coffee to buy, and it's a great way of recording every centimetre you have lost; just ensure that you make a note of the exact place where the measurement was taken for really accurate results.

What's so special about the ball?

The exercise ball has the unique quality of allowing a huge range of movement that you simply cannot achieve on the floor. For nearly all the exercises, you need use only your own body weight for resistance, and yet you can still make the same exercise very simple or extremely challenging, depending on how you position yourself. The ball work improves body shape by sculpting long, lean muscles instead of short, bulky ones. Just sitting on the ball is good for you as you lengthen your limbs and spine, whilst using countless muscles to maintain your balance and keep yourself in position. This will eventually help to improve your posture, making you appear taller and thinner. Think of it as the difference between a dancer and a body builder – you will have the grace and poise of a dancer.

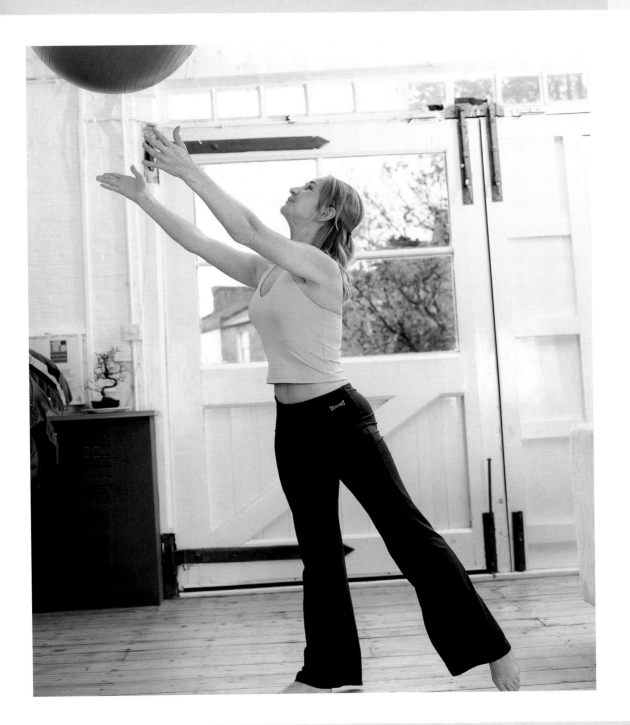

A bit of bounce

Because the ball is such a versatile piece of equipment, the book includes a section dedicated to aerobic exercise. In it you will be introduced to vigorous exercises that will raise the heart rate enough to give you a fantastic fat-burning workout. You may not think it possible to do a full aerobic workout with a giant inflated ball, but, trust me, you can. And it's a lot of fun too!

Mental and physical balance

In years gone by human survival depended on our ability to hunt down the next meal, or to protect ourselves from enemies. Today, however, survival is about achieving equilibrium, both around and within us, and improving our physical ability to balance will also help us to stay mentally focused.

Working with the ball is exercise for the body and the mind, helping us to develop

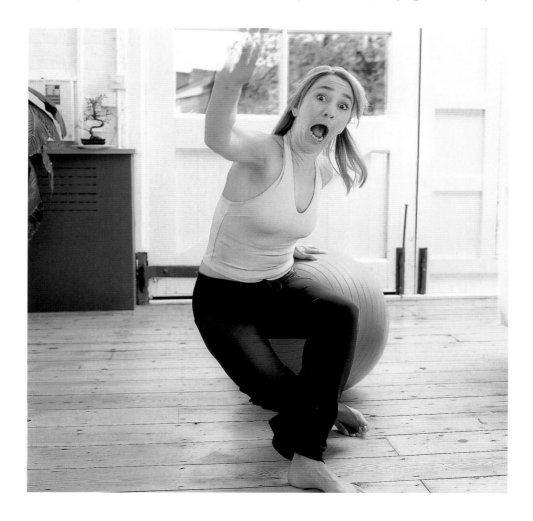

movements that develop control from within. It is not enough simply to do the movements; we must also think about how we are doing them.

In gaining control over our body we can gain control over our lifestyle. How often have you thought, 'I really didn't want to eat that chocolate bar, but I just couldn't help it'? How is it that seemingly intelligent people cannot prevent their hand from opening the fridge door and eating those things that they know they will regret later? Using this book, and with my help, you will gain both physical and mental control. You're not going to set yourself unrealistic goals that you cannot achieve as this will back up your belief that you have no control over your actions and reinforce feelings of failure. Instead, there will be significant yet manageable changes in your physical activity and diet, changes that you will enjoy and embrace as they balance your mental and physical self.

Falling off the ball at some point is inevitable, but you are never far from the floor when this happens – only around 55–65cm (22–26in), depending on the size of your ball. It is worth learning, at this safe height, how to challenge your balance and co-ordination, and how to fall with grace. Training your body to respond quickly to imbalance is a skill that could, at some time in your life, save you from a potentially nasty fall.

Me and my ball

As a very active child, who was always into gymnastics and dancing, it is not surprising that I was given a huge, orange, vinyl ball one Christmas to roll around on. I remember its smell, its texture, and even its packaging. I recall that by draping myself over it I felt the most heavenly stretches throughout my body.

Following on from my professional dance training, and finding myself in the fitness industry, I was delighted one day when I discovered a ball workshop in my area. I went along and sure enough all the old feelings come flooding back. Never had my body felt so alive as every tiny little muscle fought for balance and stability.

Looking around me, I was amused to see people whom I knew to be very physically fit in despair, wondering why they were feeling so weak in spite of their regular training routines. I knew then that the ball was the key to working the smaller muscles that are so frequently neglected by other equipment and workouts. And sure enough, today it is in gyms and rehab studios everywhere – the most treasured piece of equipment for many a personal trainer.

In my ball classes I have seen people develop a whole new attitude to exercise, helping them to grow in both confidence and stature, and I very much hope that this book will do the same for you.

CHAPTER 1: ABOUT THE BALL

A short history of the ball

The gymball – or Swiss, exercise, stability, gymnastic or flexi ball, as it is otherwise known – was first seen being used in physiotherapy circles in the 1960s in Switzerland (hence the name 'Swiss ball'). It was used there in the management and treatment of orthopaedic and neurological disorders. In particular, it was found to be beneficial to children with cerebral palsy as it helped them to develop balance skills and to maintain reflex response.

Dr Klein Vogelbach was the first therapist to use the ball in clinical applications, and on adult orthopaedic patients through the 1970s and 1980s. It was also employed extensively around this time in the treatment of spinal injuries. Physiotherapists have found that the ball's shape and mobility call on deeper layers of muscles needed for overall joint stability, balance and posture, encouraging individuals to improve body and movement awareness.

Balls are currently used to strengthen pelvic floor muscles in the treatment of incontinence. They are also employed in preparing pregnant women for childbirth and in treating any nerve damage that may be sustained during delivery.

Gradually the ball has moved out of the exclusive realm of therapy circles and into sports medicine and, most recently, fitness centres across the globe for the benefit of the general public.

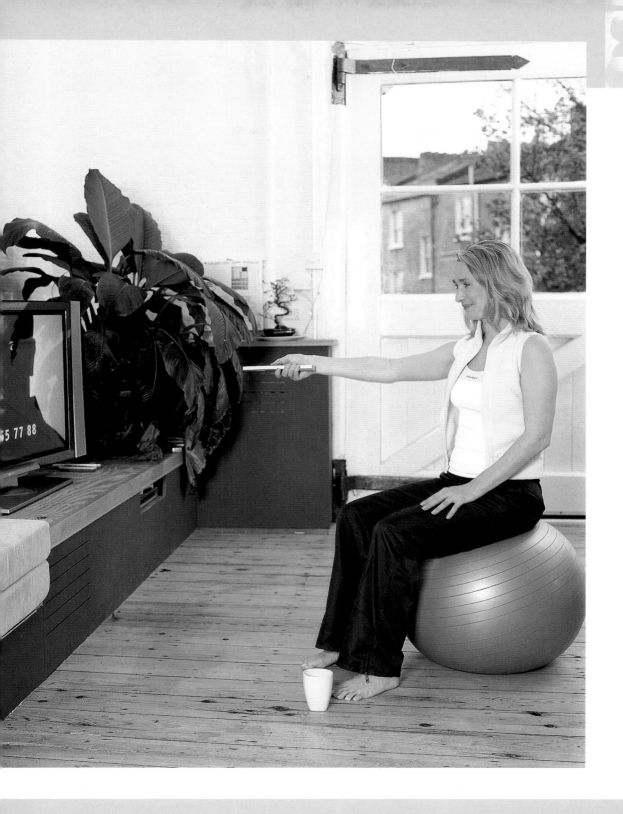

Why use the ball?

The ball is cheap, accessible and extremely versatile. It's easy to deflate whether for storage at home or to take away with you on holiday.

Unlike any other type of exercise equipment or mat, the ball has an unstable base of support so that balance is required for anything you decide to do on it. In order to balance, your body recruits many deep, stabilising muscles. These muscles are often otherwise neglected, resulting in common injuries of the knees, ankles, shoulders and the back.

With millions of us suffering from back pain, say from slouching in front of the television or hunching over a computer keyboard at work, we have to re-awaken the deep postural muscles that hold us upright. Some physiotherapists have even recommended replacing the chairs in offices and schools with balls. And this is not only to develop better posture; it has also been found that the ball can improve concentration in children, enabling them to focus for longer. In addition, studies are being conducted into the advantages of sitting on the ball for children with attention deficit disorder (ADD).

Another major benefit of the ball is in aiding and enhancing functional movement skills; in other words, the skills your body needs to meet the challenges of everyday life, such as lifting the shopping out of the car, playing with your children, or being able to reach that top shelf without pulling a muscle. Time spent exercising effectively is a wise investment and should be taken seriously.

Yoga instructors utilise the ball to aid in relaxation and to help students achieve postures that would otherwise be impossible. Pilates instructors use the ball to recreate

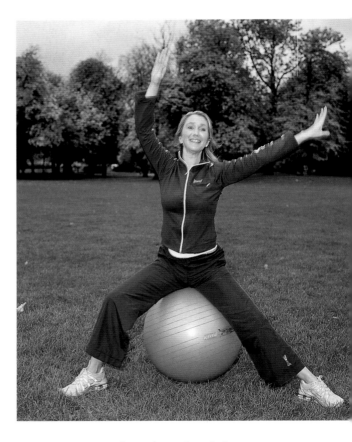

some exercises usually performed on their traditional reformer equipment. (This apparatus consists of wooden frames and a series of pulleys and springs; as it takes up a lot of space, the ball is a useful alternative.)

Perhaps most important for the purposes of this book, the ball can be used as a tool to burn calories and ultimately fat. Simply bouncing on the ball constitutes a dynamic yet safe cardiovascular workout, and you are cushioned from the impact on landing by the ball itself! As you work through the aerobics chapter (see page 22) you will notice that many traditional aerobics movements can be adapted to the ball, and they are twice as much fun when applied that way! By lifting the ball off the floor you transform it into a weight, adding a whole new dimension to your routine, whilst throwing and catching it or bouncing and circling it are guaranteed to spice up any aerobics routine.

Buying your ball

The ball comes in a variety of sizes, materials and colours and is widely available from most superstores or big sports shops. As with all consumer goods, though, some are of better quality than others. The Resources section of the book (see page 144) lists some of my preferred suppliers.

When choosing your ball, you should keep the following in mind:

- It should be made from anti-burst material as this will help the ball to retain its shape for longer. (Anti-burst does not mean that it won't burst at all, but that if it does, it will go down slowly rather than pop.)

- It should be pressure tested to around 450kg (1000lb) and should ideally have a non-slip surface.

- The ball must be the right size for your height. Most adults would need either a 55cm or 65cm (22in or 26in) ball. Generally speaking, a 55cm ball is suitable for heights of between 1.5m and 1.7m (5ft and 5ft 8in), whilst a 65cm ball is recommended for 1.7–1.88m (5ft 8in–6ft 2in). Manufactures provide their own height guidelines but these do vary. The most important factor is that when you are seated on your ball your hips should be level with your knees or higher.

- Some balls come with their own pump, whilst others have a valve which will fit a bicycle pump. If you are likely to inflate and deflate your ball frequently, my advice is to buy either an electric pump or one that is designed specifically for use with the ball (see page 144). A good way to check that you have inflated the ball to the right size is to open a door 55cm or 65cm wide, depending on ball size, and if your ball just passes through, you're away. If you are a beginner, you may find initially that you get more support and stability from a slightly under- rather than over-inflated ball.

Caring for your ball

- **Check the floor for sharp objects before you begin.**

- **Do not use the ball outdoors.**

- **Do not let animals or children play with the ball.**

- **Clean the ball with a cloth and warm soapy water.**

CHAPTER 2: BEFORE YOU BEGIN

Neutral spine alignment

Correct posture is crucial when using the ball. Your spine curves in naturally at the neck (cervical spine), then out at the upper back (thoracic spine) and in again at the lower back (lumbar spine). These neutral or natural curves are designed to absorb any shock or impact going through your body. It is only when they become exaggerated that we put unnecessary pressure on the spine, so to keep them in place you must ensure that your pelvis is also in neutral alignment – not tilted forwards or back. This is where your abdominal muscles come into play.

Think of the muscles between your pelvis and the bottom of your ribcage as a corset which, when tightened, stops your pelvis from moving in and out of its neutral position. To tighten it, imagine that you are pulling your navel in towards your spine whilst drawing up your pelvic floor muscles (these are the muscles you would use to stop yourself on the toilet in mid-flow). This is what I want you to do each time I ask you to engage your abdominal contraction.

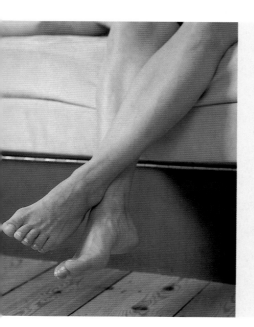

Helpful hints

- If you have any health concerns, if you are pregnant or if you are on medication or receiving medical treatment, you should check with your doctor before embarking on an exercise programme.

- Wait at least an hour after a heavy meal before exercising.

- Work on a non-slip surface – a yoga mat works well. Exercising barefoot is best, but rubber-soled trainers may be worn if you wish (and should be worn for ankle support in the aerobic section).

- Make sure you have enough space around you in all directions.

- Stop an exercise if you feel pain or discomfort whilst doing it. Always build up gradually.

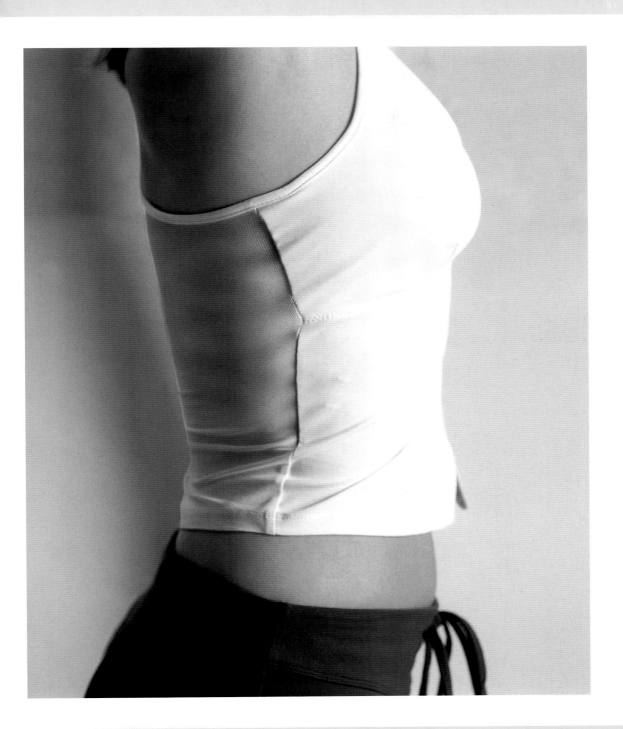

Postural set-up and awareness

To help you perform the next two exercises look at yourself side-on in a full-length mirror. This will allow you to check your posture visually, although with practice you will learn to feel instinctively if you are in correct alignment.

THE AIM:
To achieve correct posture in a seated position and to become familiar with neutral spine and pelvis.

SEATED NEUTRAL POSITION

❶ Sit in the centre of your ball, ensuring that your feet are hip-width apart, knees directly over ankles and arms relaxed by your sides. You should be sitting right up on your sitting bones (the bony bits underneath your bottom). With your shoulders relaxed, lengthen your body (through the crown of your head), drawing the crown of your head towards the ceiling. Check your posture – the three natural curves of the spine should still be in place.

❷ Engage your abdominal contraction by pulling your navel in towards your spine and drawing up your pelvic floor muscles. Keep this position for a few minutes, allowing your body to get used to the feeling of neutral alignment.

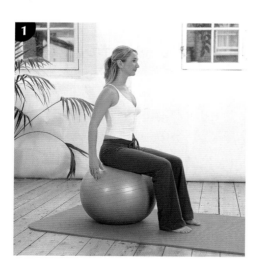

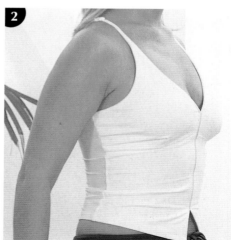

PELVIC TILTS

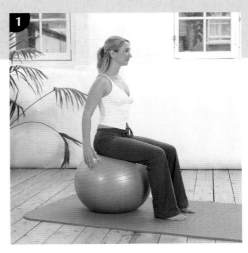

THE AIM:
To achieve pelvic mobility and to become familiar with moving in and out of neutral pelvis.

1 Start in your seated neutral position, arms by your sides.

2 Tilt your pelvis forwards by scooping in your abdominals, and drawing your tailbone under. Return to neutral pelvis.

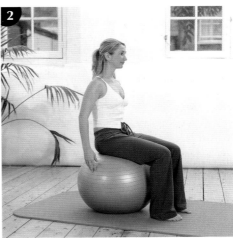

3 Tilt your tailbone back, allowing your pelvis to tilt the opposite way. Then return to neutral pelvis. Repeat 6–8 times.

Watchpoints

- **Make sure that your knees stay over your ankles throughout the movement.**

- **Do not force the movement too far.**

- **Return to seated neutral position between each pelvic tilt.**

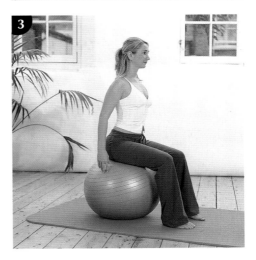

Breathing preparation

Breathing correctly is a key factor in the smooth functioning of your body. Every breath in sends vital oxygen to your cells, nourishing muscles and cleansing the blood, whilst every breath out assists in releasing toxins from your body. Good breathing can help to soothe away tension, is fundamental to stress management techniques and can help to maintain consistent energy levels. Yet so often we take shallow, laboured breaths using less than half of our lung capacity, and many people find it difficult to control and slow down their breathing when their respiratory muscles are out of condition as a result of inefficient use.

When you exercise with the ball, you need to find a natural rhythm to co-ordinate breathing with movement. Generally speaking, you will find it most natural to breathe out on the exertion phase of the movement.

When you take a deep breath, you probably automatically send the breath into the abdominal area. On the ball, however, in order to maintain an abdominal contraction for neutral spine, you need to send that breath into the back of the lower ribcage. Breathe in and imagine the ribcage expanding sideways, keeping your shoulders relaxed and down. This is known as lateral breathing.

The following two exercises allow you to explore how your breath can be directed into different parts of the body. You will be breathing in through the nose and out through the mouth, ensuring that your jaw is relaxed. Focus on your breathing and try to achieve a smooth, controlled and relaxed rhythm.

LATERAL BREATHING

THE AIM:
To establish basic postural and breathing concepts, to create an awareness of neutral spine and pelvis in a lying position and to practise co-ordinating a deep abdominal contraction with a lateral breathing pattern.

❶ Start flat on your back with your heels up on the ball. Make sure that your knees are directly over your hips and your feet are hip-width apart. Your spine should be in neutral position with just a slight curve in the lower back. Your back should not be arching away from the mat, nor pushed flat. There should be just enough space between spine and mat to slip a piece of paper through.

❷ Engage your abdominal contraction by pulling your navel in towards your spine, and drawing up your pelvic floor muscles.

❸ Place your hands on your ribcage, fingers pointing inwards. Establish a calm breathing pace, directing the breath into the back of your ribcage. As you breathe in your fingers should part, and as you breathe out they should return. On the inhale maintain the drawing-up of the pelvic floor muscles, and on the exhale re-establish the navel-to-spine action.

❹ Continue for a few minutes.

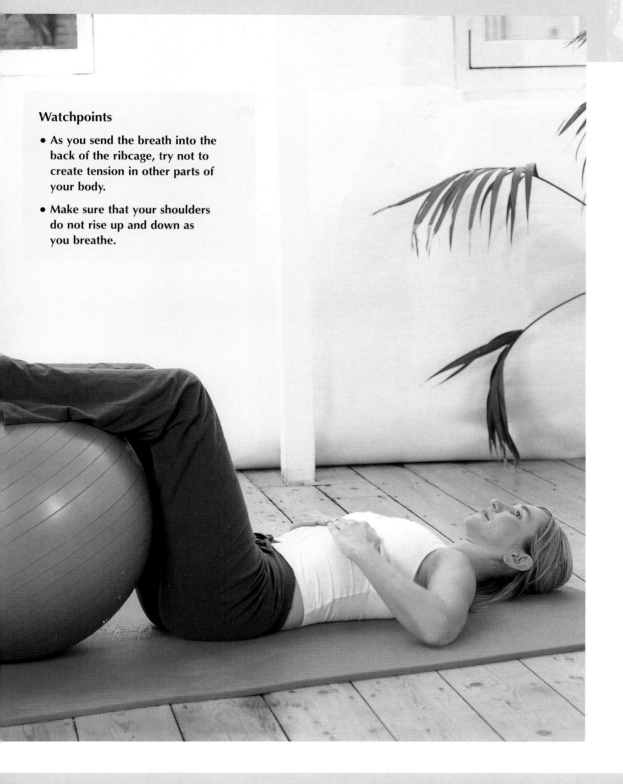

Watchpoints

- As you send the breath into the back of the ribcage, try not to create tension in other parts of your body.

- Make sure that your shoulders do not rise up and down as you breathe.

SIDE BREATHING

THE AIM:
In a side-lying position one side of your ribcage is pushed into the ball which allows you to direct your breath into the other side. This teaches you how and where to direct your breathing and also how to open up and stretch each lung and each side of the body in turn.

1 Start kneeling up with the ball on your left side and engage your abdominal contraction. Lengthen your left arm over the ball towards the floor, and allow your body to drape sideways over it. Extend your right leg out to the side, and lengthen your right arm over your head.

2 Direct your breath into the right side of your ribcage as you inhale, then exhale to release it. Take 4–5 breaths in this position, then slowly bring yourself out of the stretch.

3 Move the ball around to the other side and repeat.

Note: Before you change sides, see if you can notice a difference between the side you have opened up and the one you haven't.

Watchpoints
- Make sure that your body stays in alignment as it drapes over the ball.
- If you feel any strain in the neck, you can support your head by bending your right arm and resting your head on your hand.
- If you feel there is too much weight on your knee, try pushing your outstretched foot into the floor.

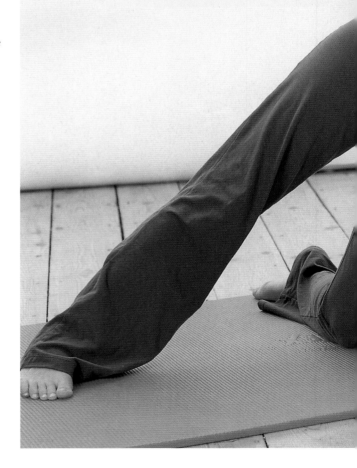

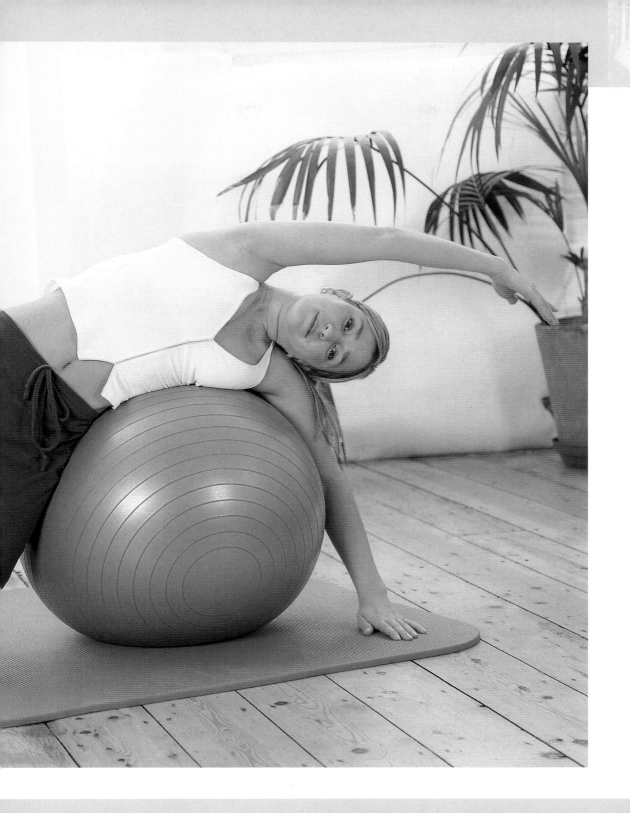

CHAPTER 3: AEROBICS WITH THE BALL

Aerobic exercise is any form of exercise that uses large muscle groups at a regular, even pace to increase the heart rate. During aerobic exercise you take in more oxygen, which helps to convert the fat and glucose that are stored in your body into energy. The aerobic moves shown in this section can be used for two main purposes.

First, the aerobics comprise a sustained sequence of movements lasting 20 minutes or more, encouraging your body to use stored fat for energy. As part of a weight-loss plan, I suggest that you try to do at least 20 minutes of aerobics work with the ball at least three times a week. If you combine this with the toning exercises that follow and my healthy eating plan (see page 136), you should achieve optimum weight-loss results.

Second, aerobics can be used to help you to warm up and prepare your body for other exercise to follow. If you are using this section to warm up before the toning exercises, and do not have time to do the full 20 minutes, I suggest selecting just five exercises and spending one or two minutes on each without resting in between.

There are ten aerobics exercises here, so for a complete session make sure you have a clock with a second hand nearby and spend either two minutes per exercise, or one minute per exercise, but repeating the sequence twice through. Working to music with a strong beat will help you to keep up the momentum. You should find that you are working hard enough to break out in a sweat, but not so hard that you can't catch your breath.

NOTE: Always build up slowly and work only to your own ability.

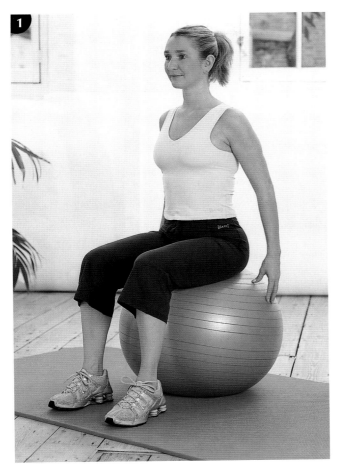

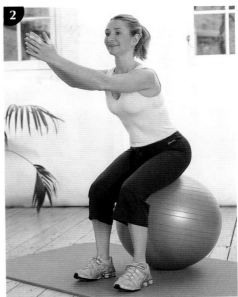

Watchpoints

- **Keep your knees directly over your ankles when bouncing.**
- **Make sure that you do not bend or twist the spine as you bounce.**

BOUNCING ON THE BALL

❶ Start seated on the ball with your feet hip-width apart, knees directly over your ankles and arms by your sides. Push your feet into the floor to start yourself bouncing up and down, allowing your bottom to come just slightly off the ball, but not so far that the ball rolls away. Bounce gently at first, increasing in vigour as your confidence grows. Keep up your breathing and stay relaxed as you bounce.

TO PROGRESS:

❷ Start yourself off bouncing as before, then clap your hands in front of you at eye level and behind your back as you continue to bounce.

HALF STAND-UPS

❶ Start seated on the ball with your feet hip-width apart, knees directly over your ankles, arms down by your sides. Push your feet into the floor, activating your thigh muscles as if you are going to stand up, but come up only enough for your bottom to lift 2.5cm (1in) from the ball, then sit back down.

❷ As you lift up, raise your arms to eye level, then relax them down as you sit down again.

TO PROGRESS:

❸ Perform the exercise as before, only this time clap your hands above your head.

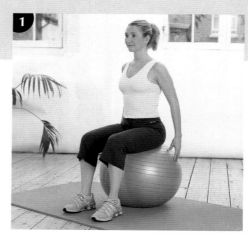

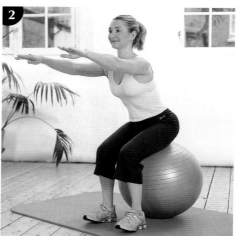

Watchpoints

- **Make sure that your knees do not come in front of the line of your ankles.**

- **Remember to keep your abdominal contraction engaged so that your spine stays fixed in its neutral position.**

- **Do not lift so far off the ball that it can roll out from underneath you.**

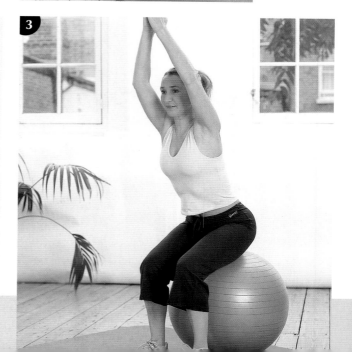

FOOT TAPS

❶ Start seated on the ball in neutral position. Make sure your feet are hip-width apart, knees over ankles, and arms down by your sides with your hands lightly touching the ball.

❷ ❸ Step your right foot out to the side, taking your weight on to it, then lightly tap your left foot in front.

⬤ Repeat on the other side, initiating a bouncing action as you move from side to side. Bounce gently at first, increasing in vigour as your confidence grows.

Watchpoints

- **Remember to keep your abdominal contraction engaged as you move from side to side, so that your spine stays fixed in its neutral position.**

- **Keep your hands in contact with the ball to help stabilise yourself.**

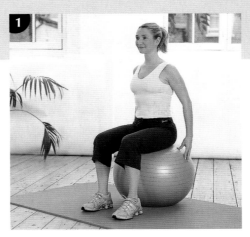

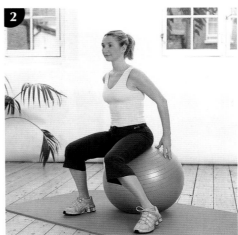

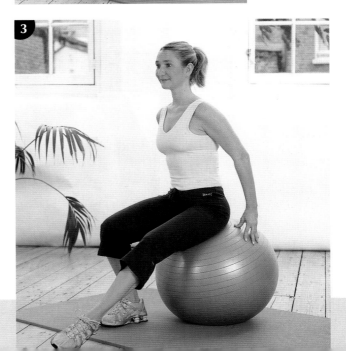

25

JACKS

❶ Start seated on the ball in neutral position, feet hip-width apart, knees over ankles, arms down by your sides.

❷ Initiate a bouncing action, extending your right arm and right leg out sideways on the first bounce and bringing them back to the starting position on the second. Repeat on the other side, keeping a steady rhythm.

Bounce gently at first, increasing in vigour as your confidence grows.

TO PROGRESS:

❸ From your neutral seated position, on your first bounce extend both legs and both arms out to the side at the same time. On the second bounce return the legs to their starting position, and bring your arms back to your sides, ready to go again.

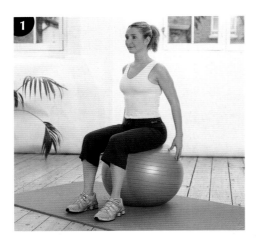

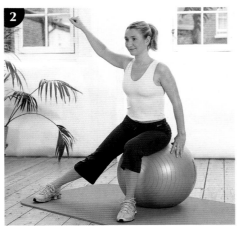

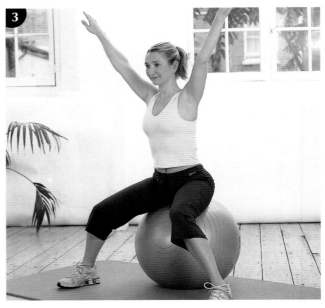

Watchpoints

- Make sure as you move your leg(s) out to the side that your knees point in the same direction as your toes.

- Keep your spine in neutral and avoid bending or twisting as you bounce.

ROCKS FROM SIDE TO SIDE

❶ Start seated on the ball in neutral position. Walk your feet out to a wide position, knees bent, turning your legs out so that your feet and knees are pointing out at a 45-degree angle (or as far out as is comfortable). Push forwards into the hips so that your weight is right at the front of the ball.

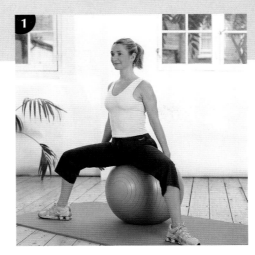

❷ Push your weight over on to your left leg so that your left knee is bent and your right leg is extended. Make sure that your left knee stays directly over your left ankle. By pushing into the floor and activating the left thigh muscle, push yourself all the way over to the other side. You should now have your right knee bent and your left leg straight. Continue to push from side to side, allowing the ball to roll underneath you.

TO PROGRESS:

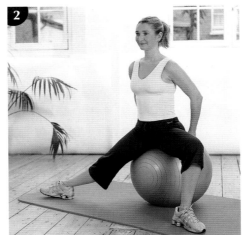

❸ Start your rocks from side to side as before. As your left leg bends, move your arms across your body so that they are pointing towards your outstretched right leg. As you move across the ball bending your right leg, move your arms across the body to point now towards your extended left leg. Keep moving from side to side in a steady rhythm.

Watchpoints

- **As you move from side to side, keep your weight at the front of the ball so that your legs work hard.**

- **Make sure that your spine does not twist as the arms move.**

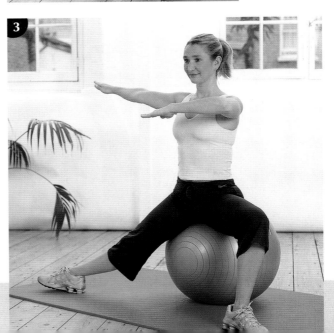

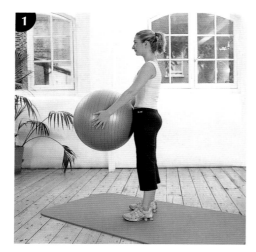

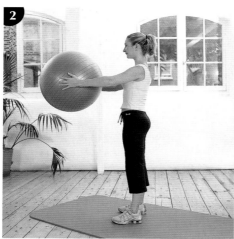

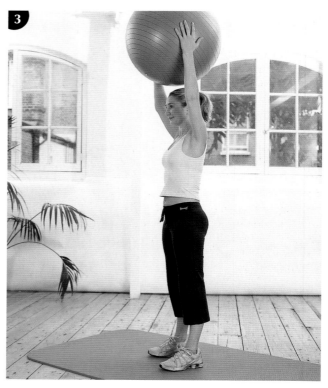

Watchpoints

- **As your arms move up and down, keep your abdominal contraction engaged throughout, so that your spine stays fixed in its position.**

- **Elbows should be slightly relaxed to avoid jarring the elbow joint.**

ARM RAISES

❶ Stand in neutral position and engage your abdominal contraction. Your feet should be hip-width apart and your knees slightly relaxed. Hold the ball in front of you, resting it against your thighs.

❷ Keeping your arms straight, with elbows just slightly relaxed, raise the ball to chest height.

❸ After a second, raise it up above your head, then lower it, first to chest height and hold the position for a second, then all the way down to your starting position. Repeat, keeping a steady rhythm.

SQUATS

1 Stand in neutral position and engage your abdominal contraction. Your feet should be hip-width apart, knees slightly relaxed. Hold the ball in front of you with your arms relaxed down.

2 Bend your knees and sit back (as though you were sitting in a chair), and at the same time bring the ball forwards to chest height. Straighten your knees, bringing yourself back to your starting position, and at the same time lower the ball back down. Repeat, keeping a steady rhythm.

TO PROGRESS:

3 Start as above. As you sit back into the squat, this time raise your arms up until they are just above your forehead. Straighten your knees, bringing yourself back to your starting position, lowering your arms back down.

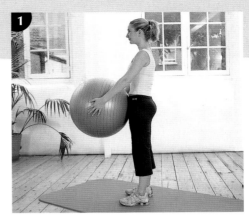

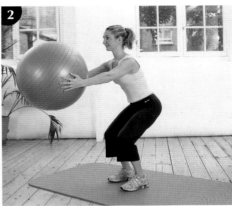

Watchpoints

- **Do not bend your knees more than 90 degrees.**

- **As you bend, keep your knees directly over your ankles and make sure that they stay hip-width apart.**

- **Remember to keep your abdominal contraction engaged as you squat, so that your spine stays fixed in its neutral position, ensuring that you do not arch the lower back.**

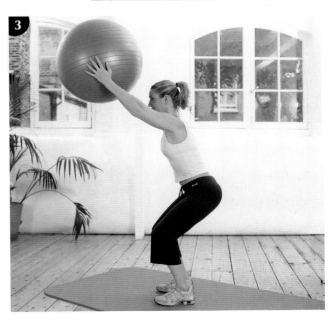

PENDULUM SWINGS

❶ Stand with your feet wider than hip-distance apart and your legs slightly turned out. Hold the ball in front of you, arms relaxed down.

❷ Bend your knees and swing the ball all the way up to head level on the right side, whilst transferring your weight on to your right leg and lightly tapping your left foot on the floor.

❸ Swing the ball all the way down, bending your knees as it passes the centre.

❹ Transferring your weight to your left leg, reach the ball up to your left side. Swing from side to side, keeping a steady rhythm.

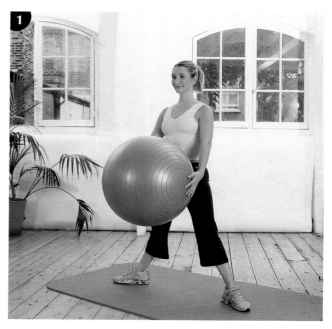

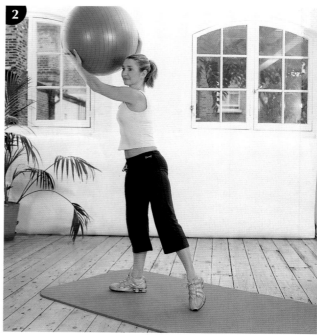

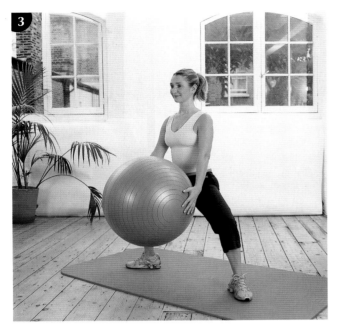

Watchpoints

- Bend your knees as the ball passes the centre, keeping ankles over knees and knees over the line of your feet.

- Make sure that you do not bend lower than 90 degrees.

- Keep your arms relaxed as they swing from side to side.

- Avoid twisting your spine, as you reach your arms up.

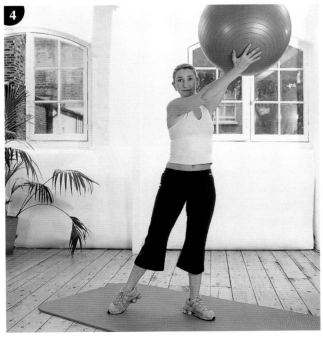

SINGLE ARM CIRCLES

❶ Stand in neutral position, with your feet together and the ball overhead.

❷ ❸ Take a step to the side with the right foot, bending the knees, then put your feet back together by joining the left foot to the right. At the same time circle your arms to the left, going full circle to where you started above your head. Repeat on the other side, working your arms and legs in unison, then continue alternating sides

TO PROGRESS:

❹ Start as above. Take a step to the right side and circle your arms to the left at the same time (as before).

❺ This time, however, as you join the left foot to the right, add a little spring by pushing off the right foot, then landing on both feet. Repeat on the other side, this time springing as the right foot comes back in.

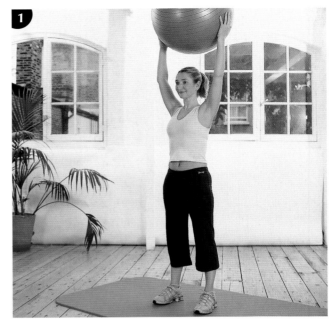

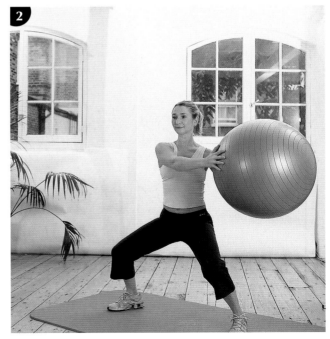

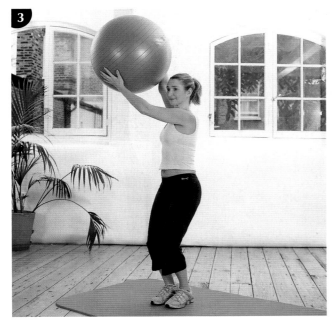

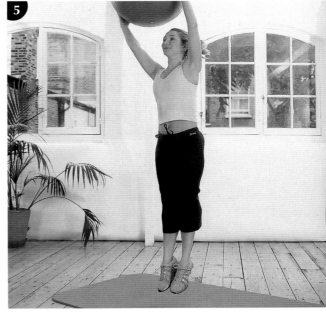

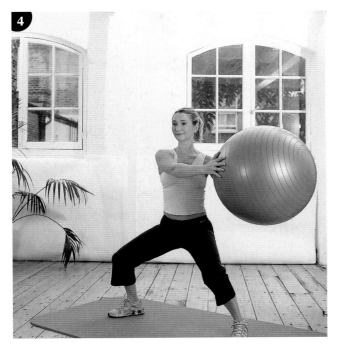

Watchpoints

- Keep your hips and shoulders square to the front as you circle your arms.

- Bend your knees as you step out to the side.

- If you add in the spring, make sure that you bend your knees as you land.

DOUBLE ARM CIRCLES WITH DOUBLE SIDE STEPS

❶ Stand in neutral position, with your feet together and the ball overhead.

❷ ❸ Step your right foot out to the side, bending the knees, then bring the left foot in, straightening the legs.

❹ ❺ Step the right foot out to the side again, bending the knees, and bring the left foot in again, straightening the legs. As you move your legs, draw two full circles with your arms, circling down to the left as you step your right foot out and up to the right as you join your left foot in.

● Repeat, coming back to the left.

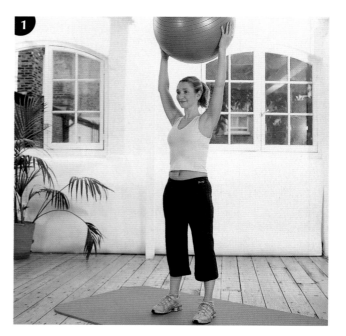

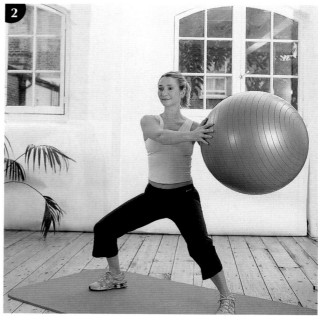

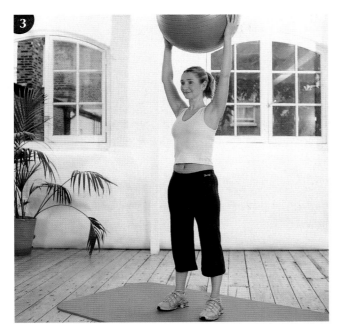

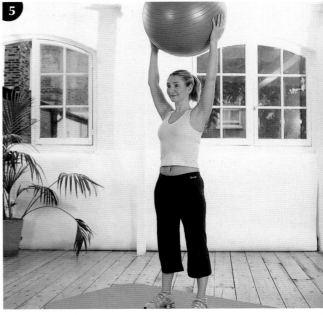

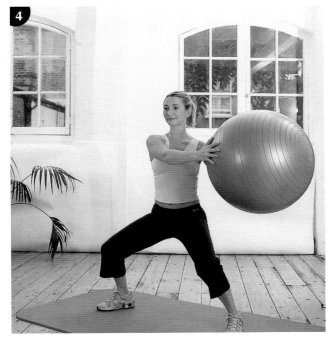

Watchpoints

- Try to co-ordinate your arm and leg movements.

- As you complete the circle by bringing your arms overhead, make sure that your spine is in neutral position.

- Bend your knees as you step out to the side, keeping them aligned with your feet.

- Keep your hips and shoulders facing the front.

In this section we will be looking at our abdominal muscles. For many of us, strengthening and toning the abdominal area is synonymous with that ultimate goal: the flat tummy. Here, however, you will be working all of the deep abdominal muscles as well as the superficial ones, so that not only will you look toned, but you will also be helping to protect your spine by strengthening those muscles that keep it in alignment – weak postural and abdominal muscles being one of the biggest causes of lower back pain.

On the ball your stabilising abdominal muscles work hard to keep you balanced whilst you exercise. This achieves a strengthening in this area that other activities and exercise regimes do not. You must remember, though, that to banish the bulge around your middle you need lots of aerobic activity too (ideally at least three 20-minute sessions a week, see page 22), so that your body has a chance to burn off the excess fat that is stored there.

The exercises in this section should be controlled and done at a steady pace. Remember to engage your abdominal contraction before performing any of the exercises and keep it in place throughout. This will avoid placing any unnecessary pressure on the lower back by keeping the spine in its neutral position. If you experience any tension in your neck whilst doing these exercises, try gently supporting your head with one hand. Any tension you do experience should lessen as your abdominals grow stronger.

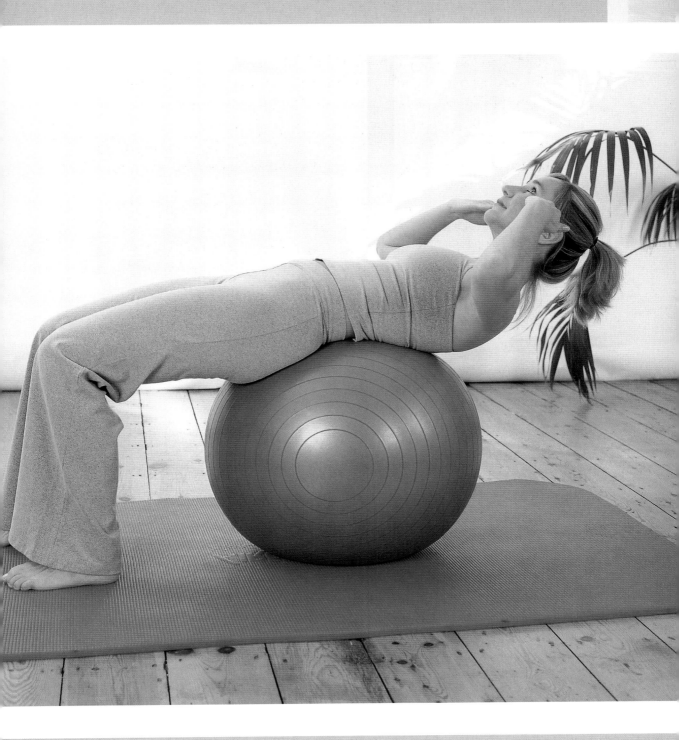

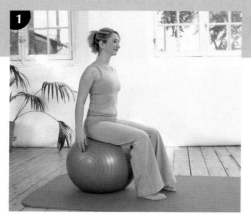

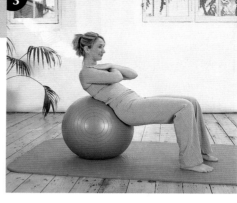

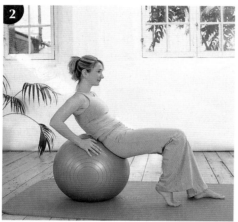

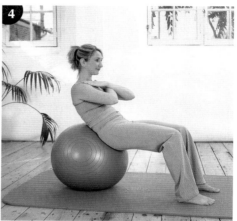

TRUNK CURLS

If you are used to doing abdominal curls on the floor, this exercise will amaze you – it really is much more challenging on the unstable surface of the ball!

THE AIM:
To strengthen your abdominal muscles.

---

❶ Start seated on the ball in neutral position, ensuring that your feet are hip-width apart and your knees are directly over your ankles.

❷ Slowly walk your feet forwards, leaning your weight back into the ball as it rolls up your spine. Stop when it is underneath your lower back, making sure that your knees are still directly over your ankles. Your shoulders should be higher than your knees, at about a 45-degree angle. This is called the incline position.

❸ Place your hands across your chest and make sure that you have engaged your abdominal contraction.

❹ Curl your upper body, drawing your ribcage towards your hips. When you have curled up as far as is comfortable, slowly take the movement back down to your starting position. Repeat 10–15 times.

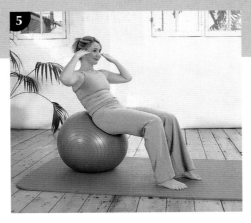

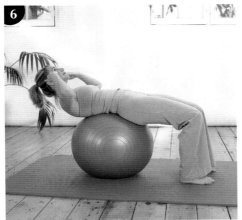

Watchpoints

- Make sure that it is your torso that is curling rather than the ball rolling. The ball should not move.

- Stay in control of the movement throughout. You should be counting approximately 3 seconds as you lift and 3 seconds as you lower.

- Try to keep your neck in neutral position throughout.

- Exhaling as you lift will help you to keep your abdominal contraction engaged.

- Do not lower yourself so far down that your spine comes out of neutral position and overarches.

TO PROGRESS:

❺ *Progression 1* Repeat steps 1 and 2 as before, only this time, to increase the intensity, perform the curls with your hands lightly touching your temples.

⬤ *Progression 2* Repeat steps 1 and 2 as before, then, once in the incline position, move your feet and knees together. This will reduce the base of support and give you more of a balance challenge as you take the curls. Choose between the two hand positions depending on how challenging you find this exercise.

❻ *Progression 3* Repeat steps 1 and 2 as opposite, then, once in the incline position, take two steps back in towards the ball so that more of your body is over the back of the ball. This is called the tabletop position; your hips, knees and shoulders should all be at the same level, giving a flat appearance (like a table, hence the name). Again, you can choose between the two hand positions. Now perform the curls in this position. You will have to work harder to curl your body away from the ball. Make sure as you lower down from each curl that you lower back only as far as the tabletop position so that your back does not arch over the ball.

OBLIQUE CURLS

THE AIM:
To target and strengthen your oblique muscles for a toned waistline.

1 Start seated on the ball in neutral position, your feet hip-width apart and knees directly over your ankles.

2 Move into the incline position by slowly walking your feet forwards, leaning your weight back into the ball as it rolls up your spine. Stop when it is underneath your lower back, making sure that your knees are still directly over your ankles. Your shoulders should be higher than your knees. Place your hands across your chest and engage your abdominal contraction.

3 Curl your upper body away from the ball, twisting from the waist so that the right shoulder comes forwards towards the left knee, then slowly lower yourself back down to the centre. Repeat 10–12 times, alternating sides.

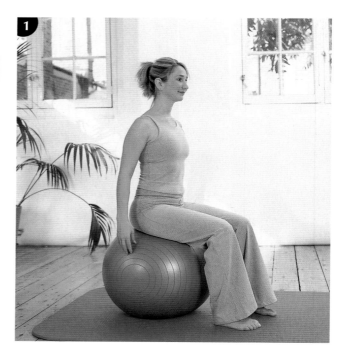

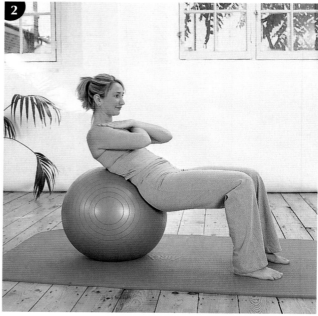

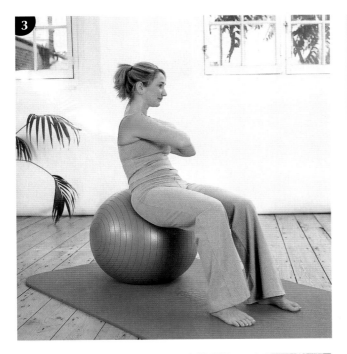

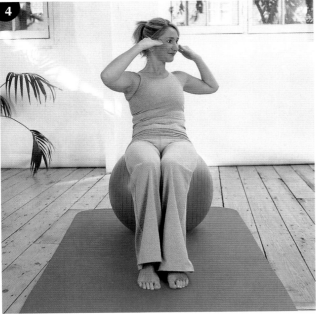

Watchpoints

- Make sure that the twist comes from your waist and not from your shoulders or elbows.

- Keep the movement controlled at all times.

- If your hands are on your temples, make sure that you do not pull on your head.

- If you feel tension in your neck, try lightly supporting your head by placing one hand behind it.

- Concentrate on keeping the ball completely still.

- Make sure that your knees stay over your ankles at all times.

- Remember to exhale on the effort, in this case as you lift and twist.

TO PROGRESS:

● *Progression 1* Repeat steps 1 and 2 as opposite, only this time place your hands on your temples and, as you curl your upper body away from the ball, twist from the waist so that your right elbow twists towards your left knee. Repeat 10– 12 times, alternating sides.

❹ *Progression 2* Repeat steps 1 and 2 as before, only this time, when you arrive at the incline position, adjust your footing so that your feet and knees are now together. You will find the balance element of the exercise much more challenging in this position. Place your hands either across your chest, or, for an even greater challenge, on your temples. Repeat 10–12 times, alternating sides.

TRUNK CURLS WITH KNEE LIFTS

This exercise is a real balance challenge!

> **THE AIM:**
> To strengthen your abdominal muscles, specifically targeting the smaller stabiliser muscles at the same time as challenging co-ordination and balance.

1 Start seated on the ball in neutral position. Make sure that your feet are hip-width apart and knees are directly over your ankles.

2 Move into the incline position by slowly walking your feet forwards, leaning your weight back into the ball as it rolls up your spine. Stop when it is underneath your lower back, making sure that your knees are still directly over your ankles. Your shoulders should be higher than your knees. Place your hands across your chest and engage your abdominal contraction.

3 Curl your upper body away from the ball at the same time as lifting your right foot about 15cm (6in) off the floor. Co-ordinate your body and leg as you lower back down to your starting position, placing your foot back on the floor. Repeat 8–10 times, alternating legs.

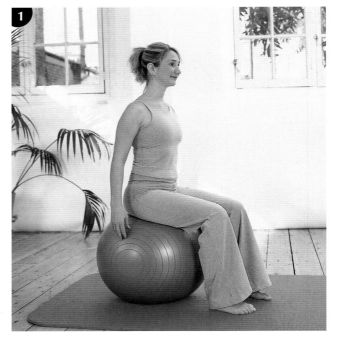

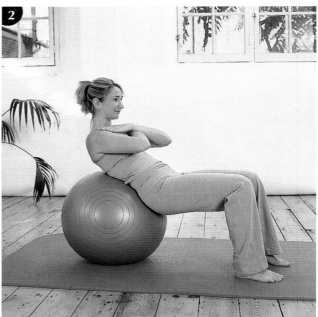

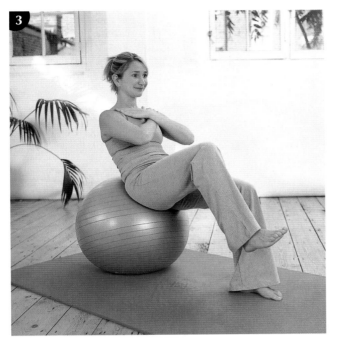

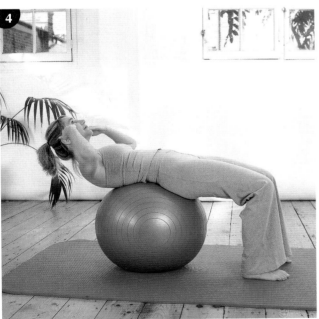

Watchpoints

- **Begin lifting your foot away from the floor as soon as you start your curl, and try to keep it off until the upper body is back to the start position.**

- **You will wobble as you perform this exercise, so always start with the most basic level and progress only as you gain in confidence.**

- **Make sure that your supporting knee stays directly over the ankle.**

- **Try not to allow the ball to move around underneath you.**

- **If you are working in the tabletop position, make sure that you lower down only as far as the neutral spine position. Do not allow your spine to arch backwards over the ball.**

TO PROGRESS:

● *Progression 1* Repeat steps 1 and 2 as above, only this time place your fingers lightly on your temples. Take the curls as before, alternating legs. Repeat 8–10 times.

❹ *Progression 2* Repeat steps 1 and 2 as above. Once in the incline position, take two steps back towards the ball so that you are now in the tabletop position. Your hips, knees and shoulders should all be at the same level. Place your hands either across your chest or on your temples. Repeat the curls, alternating legs as before. You will have to work much harder now to lift your upper body away from the ball and remain balanced.

SIDE-LYING OBLIQUE LIFTS

This exercise is great for defining the dreaded waist area and it can be done only on a round surface...like the ball.

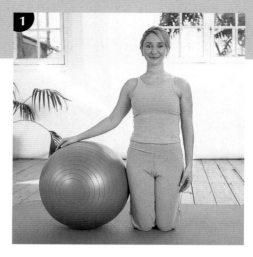

> **THE AIM:**
> To strengthen your oblique muscles, toning and shaping your waist.

1 Start in a kneeling position with the ball by your right hip.

2 Place your left hand on the ball to secure it and reach your right arm over the top until you're in a side bend. Make sure that the ball does not move as you do this. Once you are in position, make sure that your hips and shoulders are still square to the front.

3 Extend your top leg out to the side, pushing your foot into the floor to steady yourself. Place your right hand on your right temple, and keep the left hand lightly touching the top of the ball.

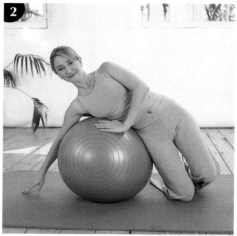

4 Keeping your hips and shoulders square to the front, lift your upper body sideways away from the ball, then lower yourself back to the starting position. Make sure you are not pushing into the ball with your supporting hand and keep your abdominal contraction engaged throughout. Repeat 10–12 times, then repeat on the other side.

TO PROGRESS:

5 *Progression 1* Repeat steps 1–3 as above, only this time place both of your hands on your temples. Perform the oblique curls in this position. You may find that you need to push your supporting foot harder into the floor to prevent slipping. Repeat 10–12 times, then repeat on the other side.

6 *Progression 2* Repeat steps 1 and 2 as above, only this time, as you extend your top leg out to the side, take it slightly in front. Then extend your bottom leg as well, taking it slightly behind. In this position your hip may need to press a little harder on to the ball than before. Then either place your underneath hand on your temple, keeping the top hand on the ball, or both hands on your temples if you want more of a challenge. Perform 10–12 oblique curls in this position.

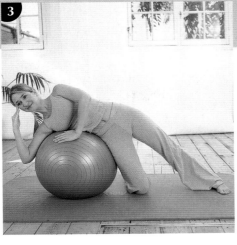

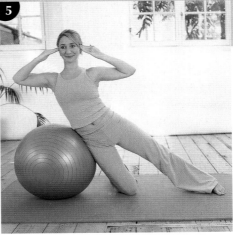

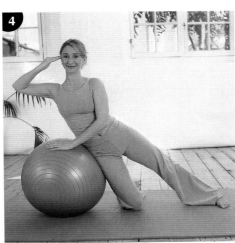

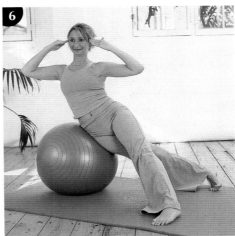

Watchpoints

- If you find the side-lying position too difficult at first, try wedging your foot or feet against a wall to keep you steady. As you gain in confidence you can then try it without the wall.

- Keep one hand on the ball to begin with. Only once you have mastered this position should you attempt to place both hands on your temples.

- As you lift up to the side, make sure that your body stays square to the front. Do not allow your shoulders to twist outwards.

- Do not worry about how high you are lifting. Just take it to a comfortable height, and as you gain strength you will find that you naturally start to lift higher.

- Try to keep your neck relaxed and in line with the rest of your spine.

- Exhale as you lift up and inhale as you lower.

BALL ROLLS

In this exercise you will have to work really hard on your abdominal contraction to prevent your spine from coming out of its neutral position.

> **THE AIM:**
> To strengthen your abdominal muscles and upper body.

❶ Start on your knees with the ball on the floor in front of you, and sit back on your heels. Link your fingers together and place your hands on the ball at chest height.

❷ Come back up on to your knees as you roll the ball forwards, allowing it to roll up your forearms to your elbows, pushing your weight into the ball until your body is in a straight diagonal line. Do not allow your back to arch; keep your abdominal contraction engaged to avoid this. Roll the ball back in, returning yourself to the starting position. Repeat 6–8 times.

Watchpoints

- Remember to engage and maintain your abdominal contraction all the way through this exercise so that your spine stays in its neutral position as you roll out.

- If you feel unable to maintain the neutral spine position, roll out only to half way, then gradually increase as you gain in strength and confidence.

- As you roll out, the ball should be touching only your elbows. Make sure your chest does not collapse on to the ball.

- Focus on the strength of the movement coming from your abdominal muscles.

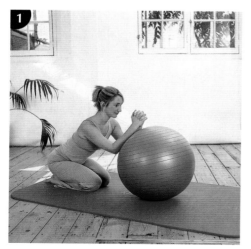

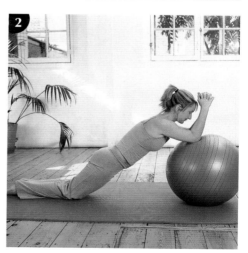

REVERSE CURLS

This one is great for flattening that stubborn part of the lower tummy.

> **THE AIM:**
> To strengthen and tone your lower abdominal muscles. You will also be working the backs of your legs to keep the ball in position.

● Start on your back, with your legs on top of the ball, arms relaxed by your sides.

❶ Walk the ball in so that it is close to your bottom, then pick it up by gripping it between your heels and your bottom so that it is a little way off the floor.

❷ Curl your knees in towards your chest, allowing your bottom to lift slightly off the floor, then slowly curl back down to the starting position. Repeat 10–15 times.

Watchpoints

- **Try counting 3 seconds on the way up and 3 on the way down, to help you to keep the movement smooth and controlled.**

- **As you curl your knees in, think about squeezing your abdominals rather than just moving your legs.**

- **Keep the ball slightly off the floor between each repetition.**

- **Make sure that you do not push off the floor with your hands. If you feel that you are doing this, try turning your hands so that your palms are facing upwards.**

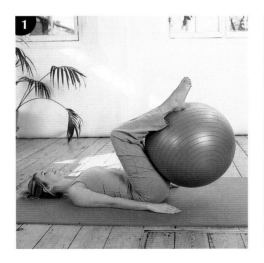

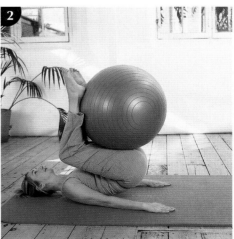

ROLL-UPS

THE AIM:
This is a Pilates exercise for strengthening and flattening your abdominal area, and for mobilising the spine.

❶ Start on your back, with your knees bent up and your feet flat on the floor. Hold the ball above your head with your arms outstretched.

❷ Bring your arms over your head, keeping them straight. As they come past your nose, start to curl the upper body away from the floor, reaching the ball in front until it is just above your knees.

● Slowly lower back to the floor, working through the spine so that you feel one vertebra being lowered into the floor at a time. Bring your arms back over your head making sure that you keep your spine in neutral and your abdominal contraction in place. Repeat 8–10 times, exhaling as you lift and inhaling as you lower.

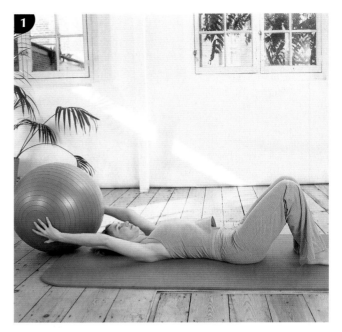

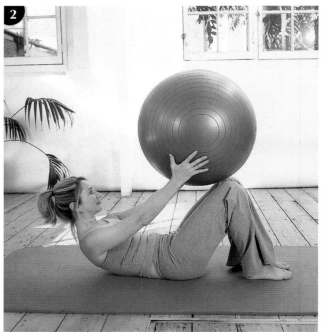

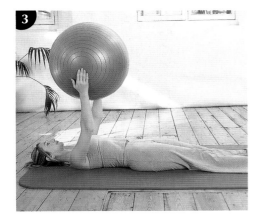

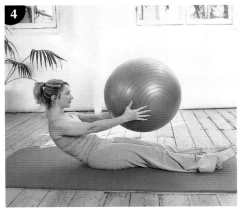

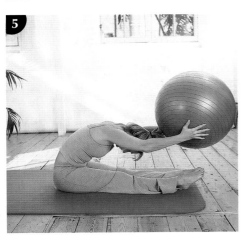

TO PROGRESS:

3 Start on your back with your legs straight, arms and ball above your head. Bring the arms up until they are at right angles to your chest and inhale as you do this.

4 Exhale, as you slowly curl up to sitting, peeling one vertebra off the floor at a time. Keep the ball at chest level.

5 As you get to the top, inhale as you reach the ball towards your toes, into a forward stretch. Exhale as you reverse the movement, rolling the spine back down into the floor, one vertebra at a time. Control the movement, and, when your shoulder blades reach the floor, float the ball back overhead. Repeat 6–8 times.

Watchpoints

- **Try to work at the same speed throughout.**

- **If you have lower back pain, stick with the basic level, keeping your knees bent.**

- **Try to keep the ball off your body throughout to add some resistance and make your abdominals work harder.**

- **If you find in the progression that you need to lift your feet away from the floor or heave yourself up, you should go back to the basic level until you build the strength to come up smoothly.**

BEND AND EXTEND

> **THE AIM:**
> To tone your abdominal muscles, hip flexors and inner-thigh muscles.

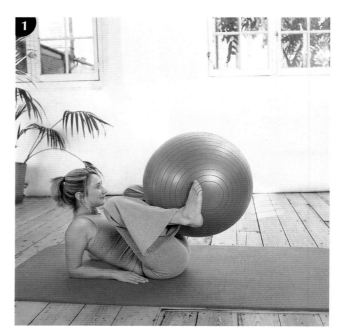

❶ Start on your back with your knees bent up and your feet flat on the floor. Pick up the ball between your ankles, squeezing tight to keep it there. Prop yourself up on to your elbows and bend your knees in towards your chest, keeping the ball off the floor.

❷ Extend your legs at a 45-degree angle (or higher). Keep your abdominal muscles pulled in tight to stop your lower back from arching as your legs extend, then bend your knees back in towards your chest, keeping a tight grip on the ball. Repeat 8–10 times, counting 3 seconds as you extend and 3 as you bend.

TO PROGRESS:

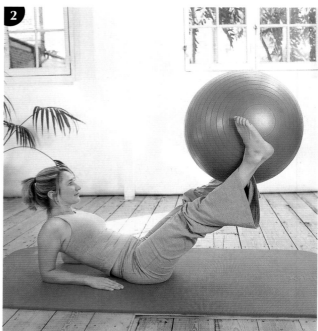

❸ Repeat step 1 as before, then extend your legs away from you at a 45-degree angle, and hold it there. Keeping your legs straight, twist the ball to the right, back to the centre, then to the left and back to the centre. Repeat 3 times to each side, then bend your knees back in. Repeat 4–6 times.

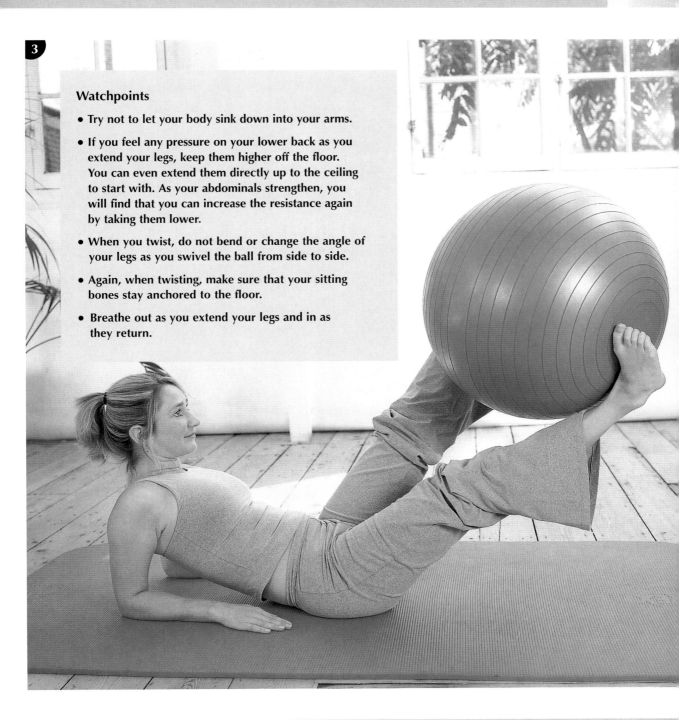

3

Watchpoints

- Try not to let your body sink down into your arms.

- If you feel any pressure on your lower back as you extend your legs, keep them higher off the floor. You can even extend them directly up to the ceiling to start with. As your abdominals strengthen, you will find that you can increase the resistance again by taking them lower.

- When you twist, do not bend or change the angle of your legs as you swivel the ball from side to side.

- Again, when twisting, make sure that your sitting bones stay anchored to the floor.

- Breathe out as you extend your legs and in as they return.

CHAPTER 5: LEGS AND BOTTOM

The exercises in this section are aimed at strengthening and toning your legs and bottom, as I am sure many of you will be pleased to hear! You will not need to bother with any additional equipment as your own body weight and the resistance of the ball are an extremely effective combination: the ball can be used as a spring to push against, a weight to lift, and a prop to roll up and down, or in and out. You will isolate, strengthen and stretch the muscles in your legs and bottom, making an amazing difference; even the smaller stabiliser muscles have to work to keep you balanced on the ball, giving you stronger, less injury-prone joints and long, lean, shapely legs.

The key to working with the ball, as in the previous routines, is to keep every movement under conscious control. It is when you work too fast that momentum takes over the movement. The exercise will become easier but less effective as it gains speed, also putting you at a much greater risk of injury. Working on an unstable surface means that your centre of gravity is constantly changing, and the only way to remain balanced is to focus on precise movements that you could stop or start at any point throughout the exercise.

One of the aims here is to produce longer muscles rather than short, bulky ones. This can be achieved by lengthening your limbs away from you as you work. Try this little exercise as an example: stand up with your feet together; lift your right leg off the floor in front of you, keeping it straight until your heel is at knee height. Now try it again, only this time, as you lift, imagine that someone is pulling your heel away from your body, stretching your leg to double its length. You should notice that, as you visualise this, your leg will float up a lot more easily than it did the first time. This is because rather than using only the big muscle in your thigh, you are now employing other muscles to help with the movement.

If you were to do the exercise the first way repeatedly over an extended period, you would probably end up with a big, chunky thigh muscle; do it the second way, however, and you will achieve a much better all-over tone in the leg. This type of visualisation will help you with all the exercises in this section.

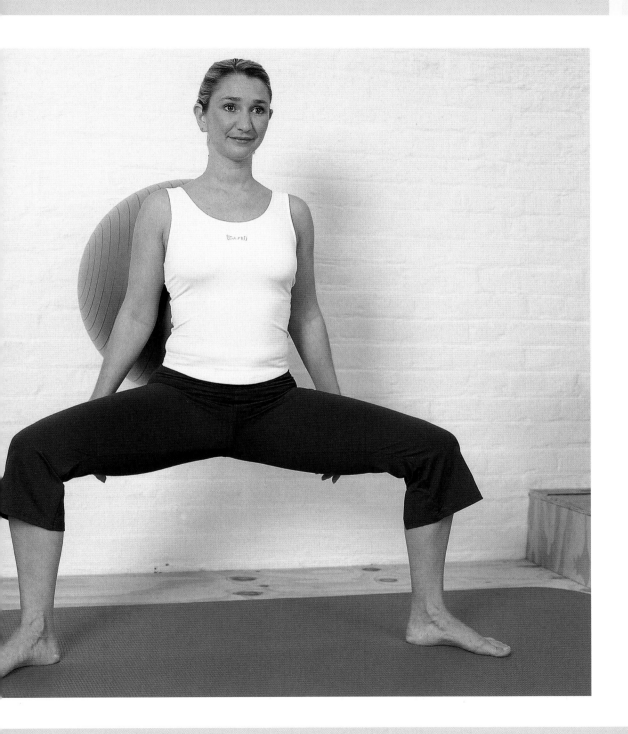

SQUATS AGAINST THE WALL

The ball provides fantastic support against the wall in these squats, helping you to keep an upright body and really work those legs.

> **THE AIM:**
> To tone and strengthen the leg and bottom muscles.

❶ Stand with your feet hip-width apart and place the ball between your lower back and the wall. Take two steps away from the wall, allowing your weight to lean back into the ball.

❷ Bend your knees, keeping your heels on the floor, until your knees are bent at a 90-degree angle or higher. Make sure that your ankles do not come in front of your toes; if they do, take another step away from the wall. Push your heels into the floor as you straighten your knees, returning to your starting position. Repeat 10–12 times, counting 3 seconds as you go down, then 3 as you come up. For a real challenge, try holding the last one down for 30 seconds.

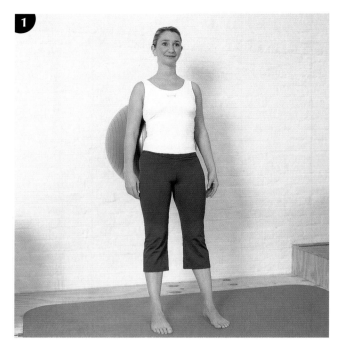

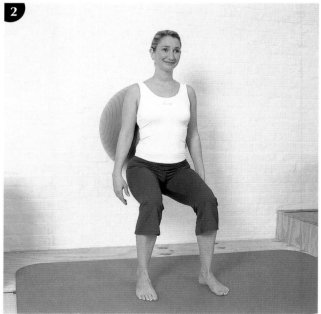

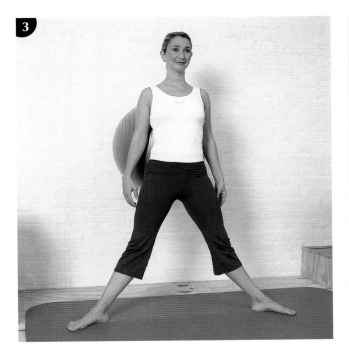

3

Watchpoints

- As you sit down into the squat, do not allow your tailbone to wrap around the ball. Remember to keep your abdominal contraction engaged so that your spine stays fixed in its neutral position.

- When you are taking the wide-leg squat, ensure that you have turned out the legs from the hip socket and not from the knee joint or the ankle.

- Make sure that there is no movement in your torso as you bend and straighten your legs; keep good posture at all times.

- Avoid any rolling of your ankles; your feet and knees should always be aligned.

- Breathe out on the effort, which in this exercise is as you straighten your legs.

TO PROGRESS:

❸ Place the ball back into position between your lower back and the wall. This time take your feet out wider than shoulder distance apart and turn your legs out slightly from your hips.

❹ Again bend your knees as before. In this position make sure that your knees are in line with your feet and that they do not roll in front of your toes. Push your heels into the floor as you return to your starting position. Repeat 10–12 times. Try counting as in step 2 opposite.

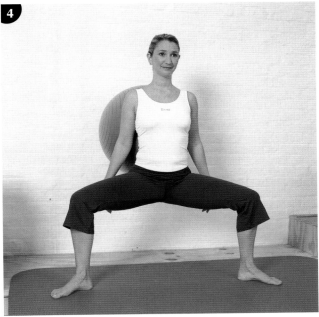

4

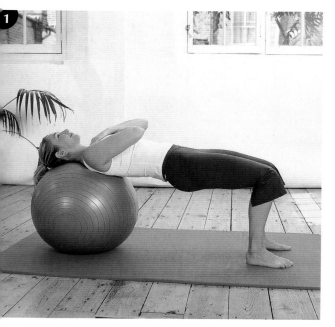
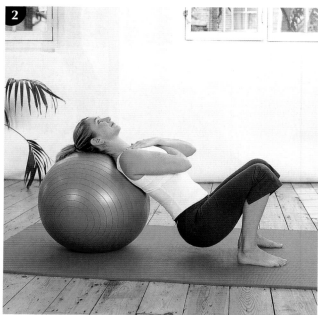

SQUATS ON THE BALL

❶ Start seated on the ball in neutral position, then walk yourself out, allowing the ball to roll up your spine, as you lie back on to the ball. Keep walking until the ball is underneath your shoulder blades and the back of your head is resting on it. Your knees should be directly over your ankles, and your hips lifted so that they are level with your knees. Cross your hands over your chest.

❷ Drop your hips towards the floor, sitting yourself into the squat. Make sure your knees stay directly over your ankles.

● Push your feet into the floor and lift your hips, returning to your starting position. Make sure that you do not roll too far back on to the ball and straighten your legs. Just push back until your knees are directly over your

THE AIM:
To work your legs and bottom muscles using the rolling action of the ball to imitate a leg press motion.

ankles again. Repeat 10–15 times. When you have finished, slowly walk yourself back up to the seated neutral position.

TO PROGRESS

❸ Repeat steps 1 and 2 as above, then, as you push back to your starting position and lift your hips, lift one foot a little way off the floor. Repeat the squat, placing both feet on the floor as you sit down again, and as you push back this time lift the other leg. Repeat 10–12 times, alternating legs. When you have finished, slowly walk yourself back up to the seated neutral position.

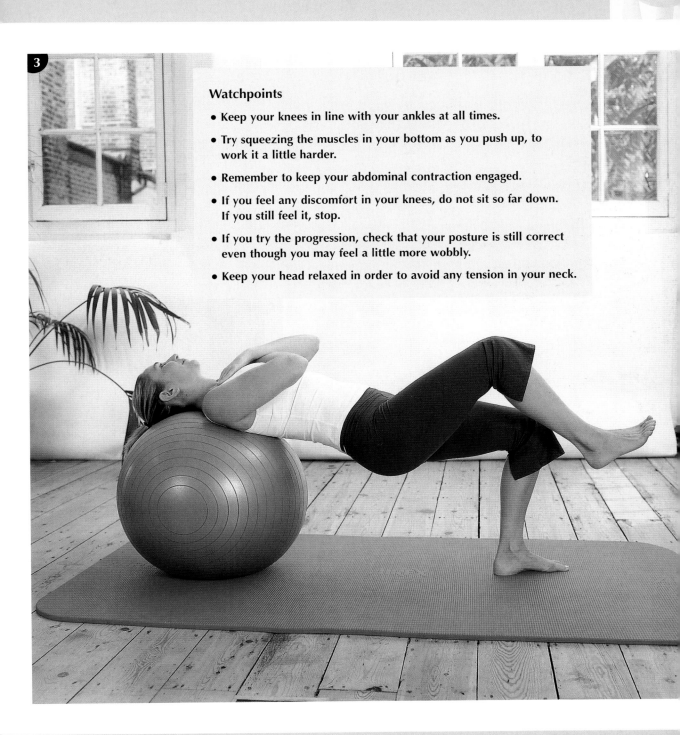

3

Watchpoints

- Keep your knees in line with your ankles at all times.

- Try squeezing the muscles in your bottom as you push up, to work it a little harder.

- Remember to keep your abdominal contraction engaged.

- If you feel any discomfort in your knees, do not sit so far down. If you still feel it, stop.

- If you try the progression, check that your posture is still correct even though you may feel a little more wobbly.

- Keep your head relaxed in order to avoid any tension in your neck.

BOTTOM SQUEEZES

❶ Start seated on the ball in neutral position. Walk yourself out, allowing the ball to roll up your spine, then gradually lie back on to the ball. Keep walking until the ball is underneath your shoulder blades and the back of your head back is resting on it. Allow your arms to relax down towards the floor. Make sure that your knees are over your ankles and your hips are level with your knees.

❷ Squeeze the muscles in your bottom hard, allowing your hips to lift slightly higher as you do so. Relax the muscles, allowing your hips to lower to knee height again. Repeat 10–15 times, then slowly walk yourself all the way back up to your seated neutral position.

THE AIM:
To add definition and tone to your bottom muscles.

Watchpoints

- Make sure that your knees are aligned over your ankles at all times.

- When you squeeze your bottom, your hips should lift naturally; do not try to lift too high as this will cause your back to arch.

- Alternate the speed by taking some long, slow squeezes, then some smaller, quicker ones.

- Keep your head relaxed throughout to avoid any tension in your neck.

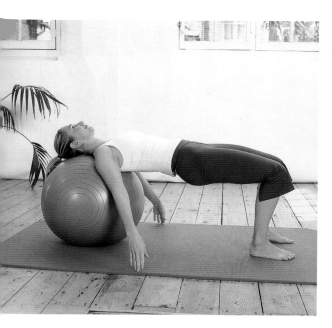

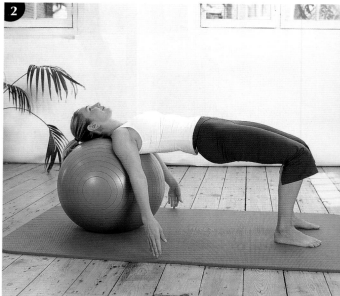

INNER-THIGH SQUEEZES

In this exercise you use the ball to push against like a spring, enabling you to work those inner-thigh muscles really hard.

❶ Lie with your feet flat on the floor and the ball between your knees in a tight grip.

● Squeeze the ball with your knees, holding for 2 seconds, then release the pressure for 2 seconds. Repeat 10–15 times, imagining that you are trying to burst the ball as you squeeze.

TO PROGRESS:

❷ Lie with your knees bent in to your chest, and the ball between your ankles.

❸ With the ball still squeezed between your ankles, extend your legs towards the ceiling, making sure that your ankles stay directly over your hips. Now squeeze the ball with your ankles as hard as you can for 2 seconds, then release, keeping your legs in the air. Repeat 10–15 times, bending your knees back in to your chest as you lower your feet back to the floor.

Watchpoints

- As you squeeze with your knees, ensure that your lower back stays flat on the floor.

- If you find it too much of a stretch on the back of your legs to lift them straight towards the ceiling, you can keep your knees slightly bent.

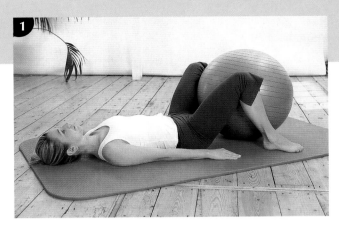

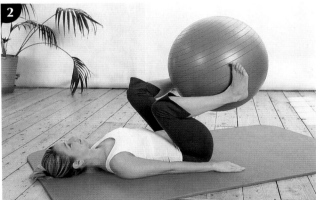

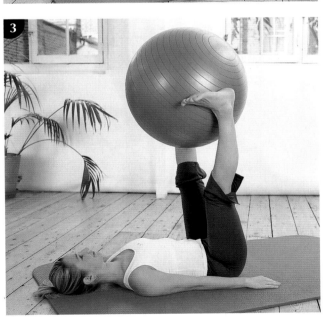

THROW AND CATCH

Just a bit of fun...although challenging all the same!

> ### THE AIM:
> To tone your inner-thigh muscles.

1 Start on your back with your knees bent in towards your chest, and the ball between your ankles.

2 Extend your legs directly up towards the ceiling, making sure that the ball stays gripped tightly between your ankles.

3 Keeping your legs extended, open them wide out to the sides, catching the ball in your hands as it drops.

4 Throw the ball back into the air with your hands, then, closing your legs together again, try to catch it with your feet. Repeat 8–10 times, then lower your legs by bending your knees in to your chest and place your feet back on to the floor.

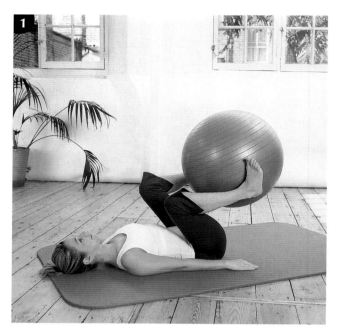

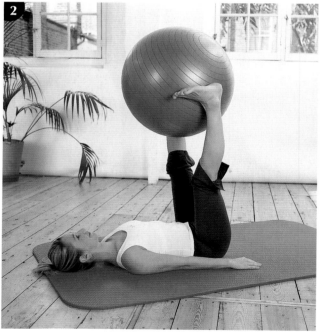

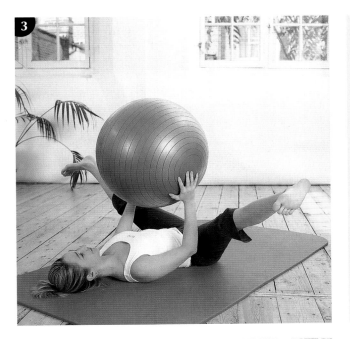

Watchpoints

- Make sure that your ankles stay over your hips throughout.

- As you drop the ball, make sure that you extend your legs out to the sides. Open them only as far as your flexibility will allow.

- Keep your head and shoulders relaxed on the floor as you throw the ball.

- If you feel this exercise in your lower back it will probably be because you have not kept your abdominal contraction engaged… pull those muscles in!

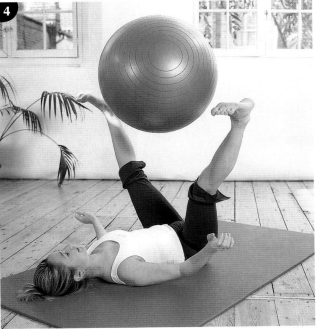

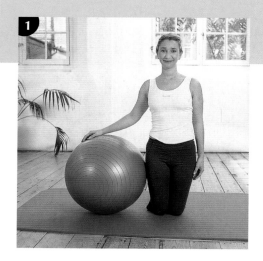

SIDE-LYING LEG LIFTS

THE AIM:
To tone and define your outer-thigh muscles.

❶ Start in a kneeling position with the ball on your right side.

❷ Reach your right arm over the ball, and extend your left leg out to the side. Make sure that your hips and shoulders are still square on to the front.

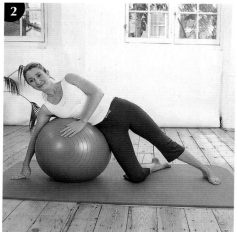

❸ Rest your left hand on top of the ball to keep it steady and raise your left leg up to the side. Keep your knee pointing forwards. Slowly lower your leg back down to the starting position, keeping it slightly off the floor. Repeat 10–15 times, then change sides.

Watchpoints

- **Do not kick your leg. Aim for slow, controlled lifting and lowering movements.**

- **Keep your hips and shoulders square on to the front.**

- **Do not try to lift your leg any higher than hip height.**

- **Try to keep the rest of your body relaxed as you perform the movement.**

- **If you feel any tension in your neck, try bending your underneath arm and resting your head on your hand.**

- **Breathe out as you raise your leg and in as you lower it.**

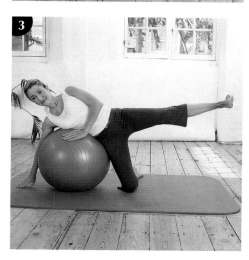

DOUBLE LEG LIFTS

The added resistance of the ball makes this traditional exercise even more challenging.

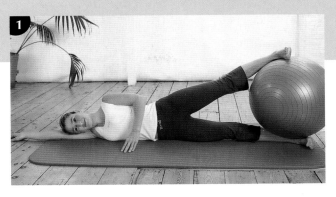

THE AIM:

To strengthen and tone your inner- and outer-thigh muscles.

❶ Lie on your right side, with the ball between your ankles. Extend your lower arm and rest your head on it. Place your left hand on the floor in front of you for support.

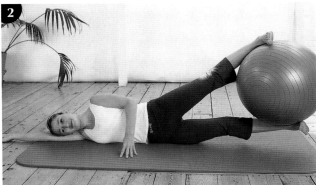

❷ Engage your abdominal contraction to keep your spine in neutral, then lift your legs slightly away from the floor, making sure that your hips stay stacked one on top of the other. Lower your legs, keeping the movement controlled throughout. Repeat 10–15 times.

TO PROGRESS:

❸ Repeat steps 1 and 2, only this time keep your left arm relaxed along your leg. You will find that without the support of your hand on the floor, this exercise becomes much more difficult. Be careful that your hips and shoulders stay square on to the front. Try not to roll off the supporting hip. Repeat 10–15 times.

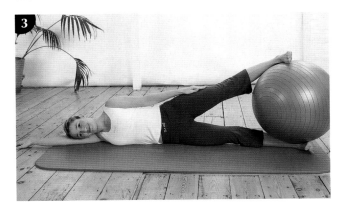

Watchpoints

- **Do not try to lift your legs too high; maintaining the correct posture is much more beneficial.**

- **Try to keep your head relaxed to avoid any tension in your neck.**

- **Remember to imagine your legs lengthening away from your body as they lift (see page 52).**

HAMSTRING CURLS

This exercise really works your bottom and the backs of your legs hard. You may find that you can do only a couple to start with, but don't give up – it will get easier.

❶ Lie on the floor, arms by your sides. Place your feet flat on the ball, and walk it away from you until your legs are straight.

❷ Lift your hips off the floor, curling up through the spine until your body forms a straight diagonal line from your feet to your shoulders.

❸ Bend your knees, rolling your heels in towards your bottom. Keep the straight diagonal line between your knees and your bottom by lifting your hips higher as you roll the ball in. Roll the ball back out to your starting position, keeping control of the movement throughout. Repeat 8–10 times. Lower your hips back to the floor by curling down through the spine.

TO PROGRESS:

❹ Repeat steps 1 and 2 as before, then lift your right leg slightly off the ball.

❺ Keeping your right leg extended, bend your left knee, rolling the ball in as before, then, controlling the movement at all times, roll it back out. Repeat 5–8 times, then change to the other side. To lower to the starting position, place both feet back on the ball and slowly lower the hips back on to the floor, curling down through your spine.

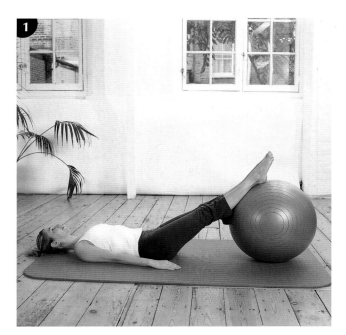

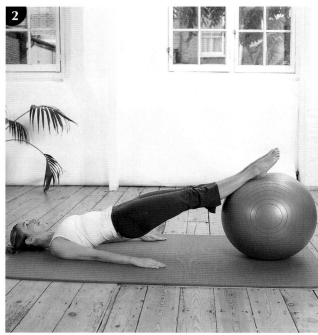

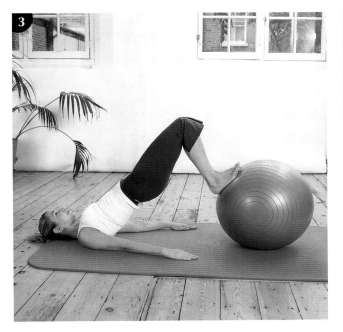

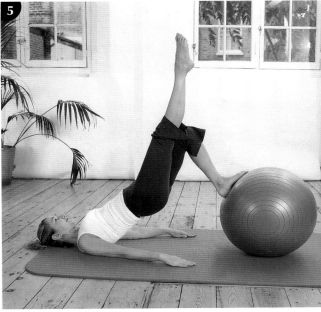

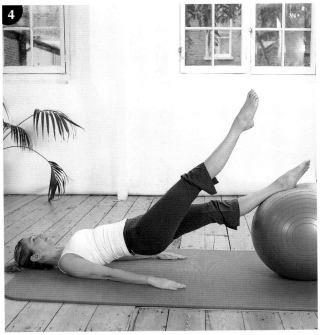

Watchpoints

- Pull the ball in by pushing your heels into it.

- Always come back to a straight diagonal line between each curl.

- Keep your feet hip-width apart to give you a wider base of support.

- Remember to keep your abdominal contraction engaged so that your spine stays in its neutral position.

- You may need to start off with fewer repetitions and build up slowly as this is a tough one.

- Try the progression only after gaining in strength and confidence with both legs.

CHAPTER 6: BACK STRENGTHENING AND SPINAL MOBILITY

Anyone who has ever had back trouble will know how dramatically a weak or immobile spine can influence quality of life, and poor posture can often be a significant contributory factor. Not only can it adversely affect the joints of the back, but it can also strain and weaken muscles and ligaments and restrict breathing. It can even make us appear much less confident than we really are.

In this chapter there are extension exercises that will both strengthen the muscles in your back, and open your posture up again: if you consider how much of your day you spend hunched forwards, whether at the computer, washing the dishes or driving your car, it is completely disproportionate to the time you spend opening out your chest or extending your spine. If your lifestyle does not naturally allow for this type of movement, you need to make a conscious effort to fit it into your regime.

This chapter also includes exercises designed to mobilise the spine so that the stiffer parts become more flexible.

Back-pain sufferers must be particularly careful doing extensions and rotations as these can aggravate a back condition if they are not performed with extreme caution. Always keep the movements very small to start with and only perform a few repetitions of each exercise, building up gradually over time. If any of these exercises causes you pain, stop immediately.

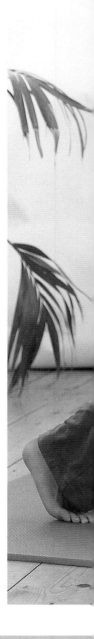

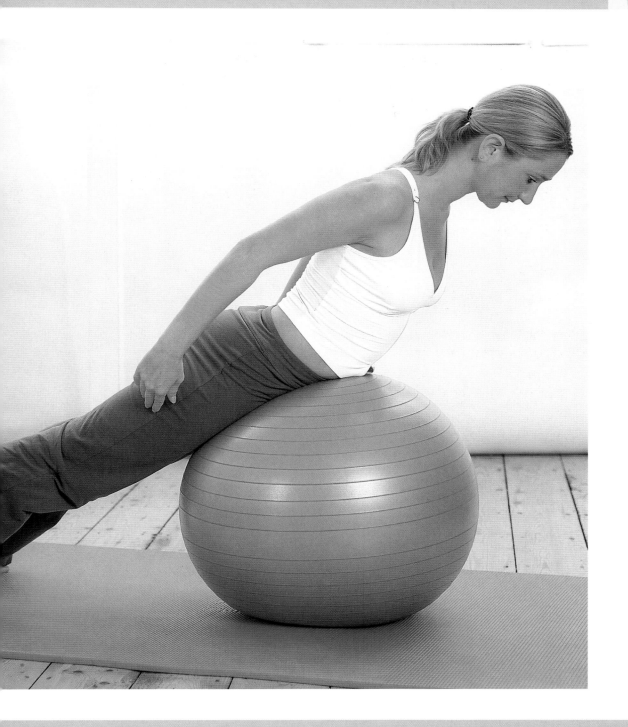

BACK STRENGTHENING AND SPINAL MOBILITY **67**

BACK EXTENSIONS

Working on the round surface of the ball gives you a much bigger range of movement than the traditional version of this exercise performed on the floor.

> **THE AIM:**
> To strengthen the muscles in your lower back and to extend your spine.

❶ Start with your hands and knees over the ball. Walk yourself out slightly until your knees are off the floor and lightly place your hands on the ball in front of you. Your weight should be mainly on your hips.

❷ Extend your upper body away from the ball until you come to a straight diagonal line. Do not overextend so that you arch your lower back. Keep your hands lightly touching the ball for support, but do not push with your arms. Slowly lower yourself back to your starting position. Repeat 10–12 times.

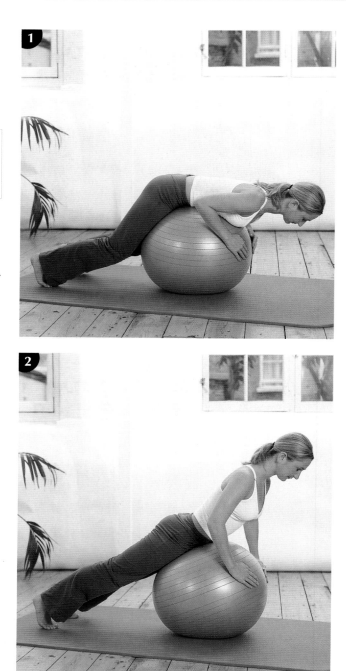

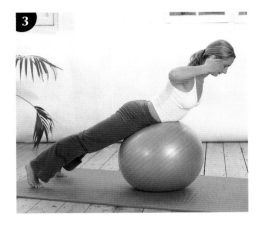

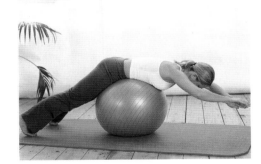

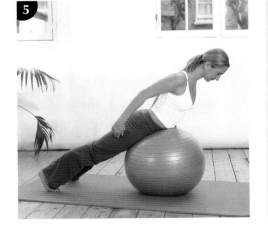

TO PROGRESS:

3 *Progression 1* Repeat step 1 as above, only this time place your hands on your temples. Extend your upper body away from the ball, until you are in a straight diagonal line. Keep your head in line with your spine, and keep your hands lightly touching your temples. Slowly lower back to your starting position, keeping control of the movement. Repeat 10–12 times.

4 *Progression 2* Repeat step 1 as above, but start with your arms by your sides. Imagine you are swimming and dive down, pushing your arms as in breaststroke.

5 As you extend your upper body away from the ball, draw your arms back, bringing them back down by your sides. Then dive down again, pushing your arms forwards, and repeat 10–12 times.

Watchpoints

- Remember to keep your abdominal contraction engaged so that your spine stays fixed in its neutral position. By pulling your navel in towards your spine you will not be able to lift up too far.

- Extend only until you are in a straight diagonal line; do not overarch your back.

- Keep the movement controlled and slow throughout.

- Be careful not to lift your head; keep your neck in line with the rest of your spine.

- Try to relax all the way over the ball between repetitions.

- Keep your feet hip-width apart for more balance and support.

BACK EXTENSIONS ON THE FLOOR

Although you have less range of movement in this version than in the previous exercise, you do have another benefit – the added resistance of the ball.

> **THE AIM:**
> To strengthen your back using the ball as resistance.

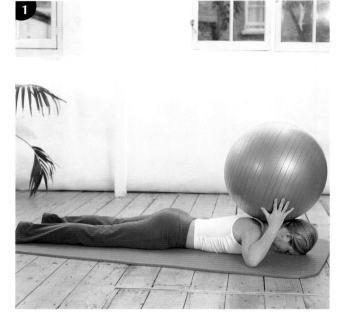

❶ Start on the floor, lying on your front. Place the ball on the back of your neck and keep it there using your hands.

❷ Keeping your focus on the floor, extend your upper body until your chest lifts away from the floor. Keep your abdominal contraction engaged – you do not need to lift very high – then slowly lower back to the floor again. Repeat 10–12 times.

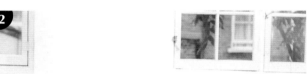

Watchpoints

- **Be careful not to lift too high.**

- **Keep your focus on the floor, making sure that your neck stays in line with the rest of your spine.**

- **Try to keep the muscles in your legs and bottom relaxed; you are trying to use the muscle in your lower back to perform this exercise.**

- **Keep the repetitions slow and controlled throughout.**

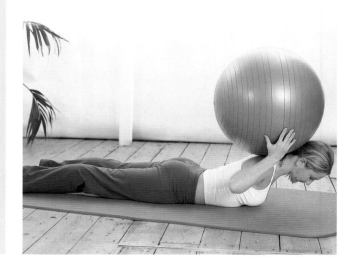

SPINE TWISTS

This exercise gives you a great feeling of growing taller in the spine.

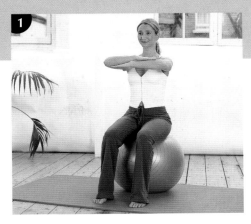

❶ Start seated on the ball in neutral position. Cross your arms in front of you so that your elbows are slightly lower than your shoulders. Make sure that you are lengthening tall through the spine.

❷ Rotate slowly to the right by twisting from the waist, keeping your hips facing the front. Go only as far as you comfortably can. Keep the movement slow and controlled.

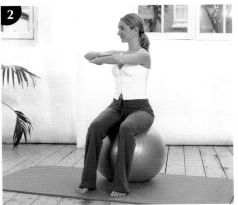

● Slowly return to the front, imagining as you do that you are growing taller through the crown of your head. Now repeat to the left. Perform 4–6 twists on each side.

TO PROGRESS:

❸ Start seated on the ball in neutral position and extend your arms out to the side at shoulder height. Imagine that your arms are being pulled in opposite directions so that you are lengthening right across the chest. Repeat the twists as above, alternating sides and ensuring that your arms stay lengthened.

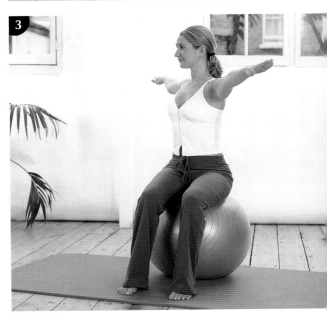

Watchpoints

- If you have any lower-back pain, keep the movements very small.

- Keep your hips facing forwards as you twist.

- Keep your abdominal contraction engaged so you feel resistance from the abdominals as you twist.

- Exhale as you twist to the side and inhale as you return to the centre.

LATERAL ROLLS

THE AIM:
To strengthen and tone your back muscles.

❶ Stand next to a wall. Place the ball between your forearm and the wall, making sure that your elbow is level with your shoulder so that your arm is at right angles with the wall. Your feet should be hip-width apart, knees slightly relaxed and your abdominal contraction engaged.

❷ Push against the ball and roll it down the wall, drawing your elbow down until it is level with your waist. Still pushing against the ball, roll it back up to the starting position. Repeat 10–15 times on each side.

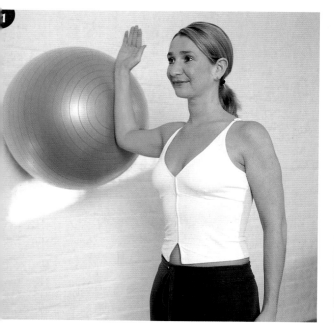

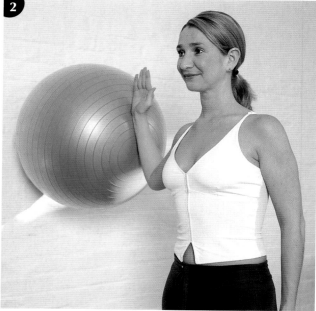

ROLLING LATERAL PULLS

1 Start over the ball on your hands and knees. Walk out on your hands until the ball is underneath your hips. Place your hands on the floor, ahead of your chest, and allow your legs to relax on to the floor behind you.

2 Press the heels of your hands into the floor, allowing the ball to roll down your body. Squeeze your shoulder blades together as you roll to focus on working the muscles in your back. You should stop when your hands are directly underneath your shoulders. You will find that your feet have naturally come off the floor. Now, pushing the heels of your hands into the floor again, roll back out to your starting position. Repeat 10–12 times.

Watchpoints

WORKING AGAINST THE WALL

- **The harder you push against the ball, the more resistance you will create, increasing the intensity of the exercise.**

- **Focus on squeezing your shoulder blades together when you roll the ball down, so that you are engaging the muscles in your back.**

WORKING ON THE BALL

- **The harder you push the heels of your hands into the floor, the more resistance you will create, increasing the intensity of the exercise.**

- **Make sure, as you roll the ball in, that your spine stays in neutral position. Do not allow your spine to collapse.**

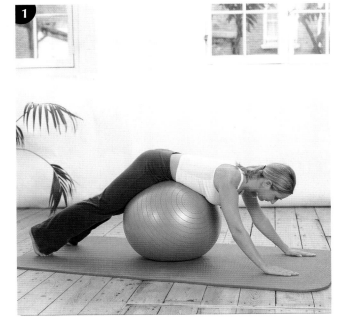

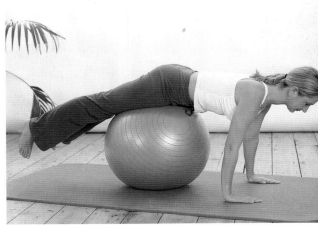

HIP EXTENSIONS

You can really mobilise your spine in this exercise by feeling each and every vertebra as it peels away from the floor.

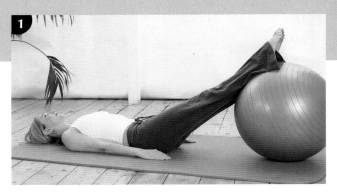

❶ Start on your back with your feet resting on the ball and your arms relaxed by your sides.

❷ Engage your abdominal contraction and slowly lift your hips away from the floor, peeling one vertebra off the floor at a time. Keep lifting until your body forms a straight diagonal line from your ankles to your shoulders, but avoid pushing up on to your neck. Slowly lower your hips back to the floor, again working through each vertebrae. Try not to allow two bones to lower at once. Repeat 6–8 times.

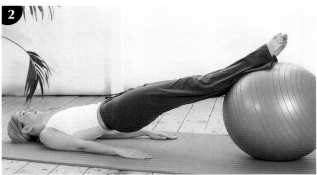

Watchpoints

- Take your time as you raise and lower your hips, slowing down further to work through any stiff areas of the spine.

- If you try the progression, you will find there is a balance challenge as well. If you are struggling, walk the ball in a little closer to your body so that it is underneath your calf muscles.

- When extending your arms overhead, keep lengthening them to the ends of your fingertips. It should feel as if your arms and legs are lengthening away from you in different directions.

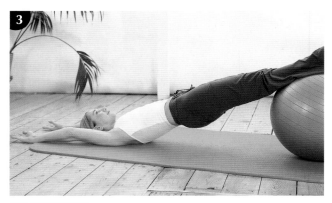

TO PROGRESS:

❸ Repeat step 1, then, with your hips lifted as in step 2, slowly take your arms over the head until they are on the floor behind you. With your hips still lifted, slowly lower your arms back to your sides. Now slowly lower your hips, working through each vertebra, one at a time, until your bottom comes back down on to the floor. Repeat 6–8 times.

ROLLOVERS

This is an advanced Pilates exercise to strengthen your spine and abdominal muscles. You may want to try it without the ball first.

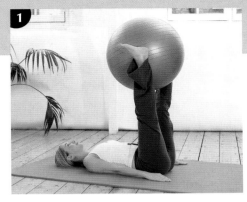

❶ Start flat on your back, arms by your sides, palms facing down. Pick up the ball between your ankles, bend your knees in to your chest and then extend your legs so that your ankles are directly over your hips.

❷ Breathe out as you peel your spine away from the floor, extending your legs over your head. Inhale as you touch the ball to the floor, then lift your legs so that they are parallel with the floor. Make sure that the movement is controlled throughout.

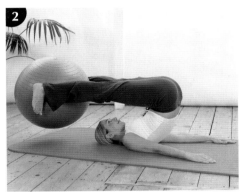

❸ Breathe out again as you roll back down, working through the spine, one vertebra at a time. Lower your extended legs as far as you can (with the ball still held between your ankles), but no lower than a 45-degree angle to the floor. Make sure that you keep your abdominal contraction engaged so that your lower back stays pushed down into the floor in its neutral position. Repeat 4–6 times.

Watchpoints

- **Try not to push your hands into the floor to help you roll your legs over. Use your abdominals instead.**

- **Do not roll over too far; avoid putting any pressure on your neck.**

- **You may place a pillow under your hips if you like, to make the exercise a little less challenging.**

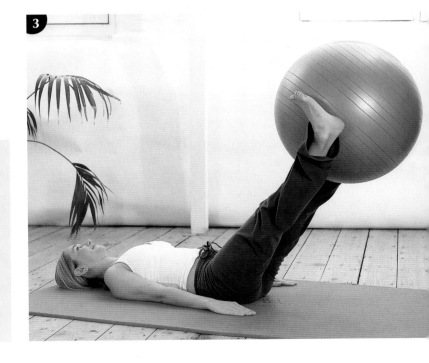

CHAPTER 7: UPPER-BODY TONING

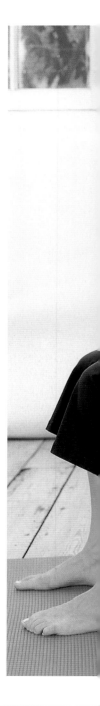

I often find that people are only too keen to lose weight and achieve a flat tummy, but are rather less enthusiastic about toning their upper body. However, exercising the body as a whole is important, as by strengthening only one area of it, you will effectively weaken the rest. There is a myth at large creating the belief that using resistance for upper-body training turns us into huge, hulk-like creatures with biceps ripping through our shirts. Well, that certainly is not the case, and as long as you use only light weights or, in this instance, the ball for resistance there is certainly no danger of you winning any body-building contests.

As well as giving tone and definition, working out with light weights twice or three times a week is a very important factor in your weight-loss programme. Resistance training will not only burn calories, but also increase your metabolic rate so that extra calories continue to burn long after your workout has finished. Working with resistance also slows the body's natural process of breaking down muscle tissue and losing bone strength and density and therefore seriously reduces the chances of suffering from osteoporosis later in life. Finally, studies have also shown that resistance training is effective at reducing blood pressure and blood cholesterol levels.

In this section we will be using the ball, our own body weight and some light weights for resistance. If you do not have any 500g or 1kg (1lb or 2lb) weights, you can use either cans of beans or the equivalent – anything you might find in your kitchen cupboard. Alternatively you can use water bottles. These work well because you can use either the big or little ones and you can adjust their weight by varying the amount of water or, if you like, sand that you fill them with. You can make yourself a whole set of variable weights in this way.

The great thing about using the ball for this section is that it even doubles as a bench on which you can perform your exercises. Of course it is a little more challenging than that, though!

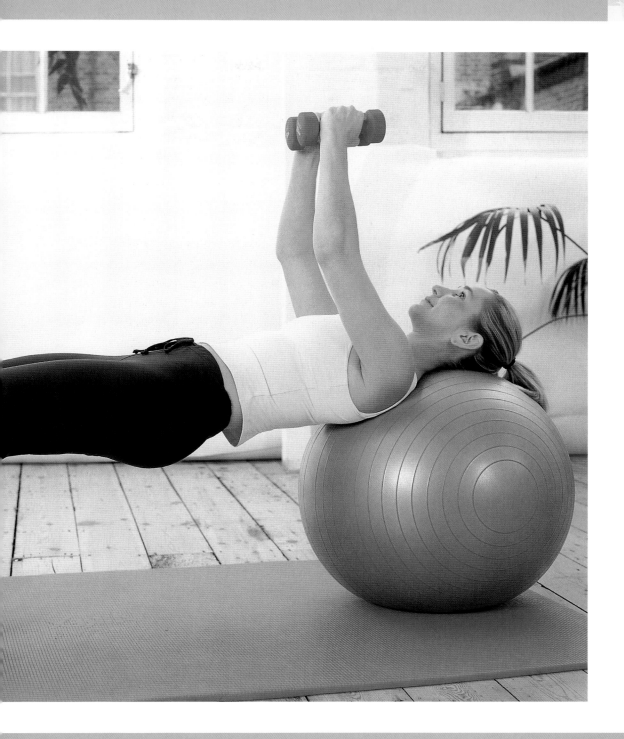

BALL SHOULDER PRESSES

THE AIM:
To tone and strengthen your shoulders and the backs of your arms, using the ball for resistance and working to maintain neutral spine position.

1 Stand with your feet hip-width apart and your knees slightly relaxed. Make sure that you have engaged your abdominal contraction and that your spine is in neutral position. Hold the ball in front of your chest.

2 Push the ball up towards the ceiling, straightening your arms. Make sure that you do not lock your elbows. Bend your arms again as you return to the starting position. Repeat 20–25 times, rest for a minute, then take another 20–25 repetitions.

Watchpoints

- It is tempting to lean back as you extend your arms overhead. To avoid this, remember to keep your abdominal contraction engaged so that your spine stays fixed in its neutral position. If you are not sure whether your spine is in neutral, check yourself sideways in a mirror as you perform this exercise.

- When lifting your arms make sure that they come slightly in front of the line of your body to avoid throwing your weight back.

- Try to create extra resistance by imagining that the ball is a lump of cement. This will prevent you from aimlessly lifting and lowering the ball without control.

- Breathe out as you lift and in as you lower. Do not be tempted to hold your breath.

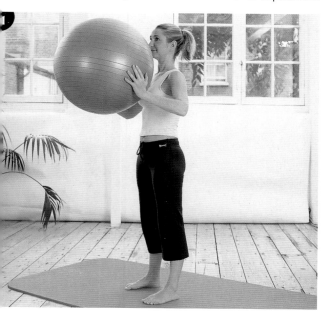

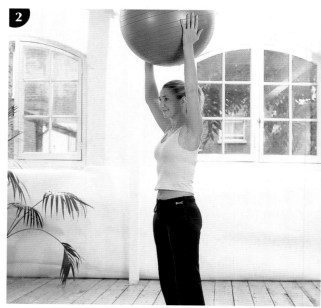

BALL FRONT RAISES

It's amazing how heavy the ball starts to feel after a few repetitions of this one!

> **THE AIM:**
> To tone and strengthen your shoulders, using the ball for resistance.

❶ Stand with your feet hip-width apart and your knees slightly relaxed. Engage your abdominal contraction, making sure that your spine is in neutral position. Hold the ball in front of you, arms relaxed down.

❷ Without leaning back, raise the ball all the way up above your head, then lower it back down to the starting position. Repeat 20–25 times, rest for a minute, then take another 20–25 repetitions.

Watchpoints

- **Keep your arm slightly relaxed so that you are not locking your elbows.**

- **Make sure that you do not allow any movement of the spine as your arms raise and lower. Keeping your abdominal contraction engaged throughout will ensure that your spine stays fixed in its neutral position.**

- **Concentrate on keeping the movement controlled throughout.**

- **Try to co-ordinate your breathing and movement to avoid holding your breath. Breathe out as you raise your arms and in on the lowering phase of the movement.**

- **Imagine that the ball is a lot heavier than it is to create your own resistance. This will increase the intensity of the exercise.**

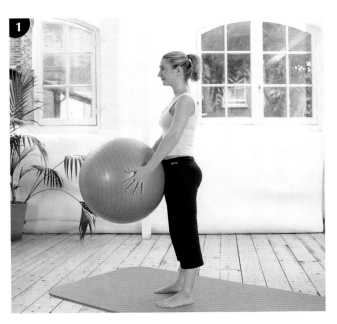

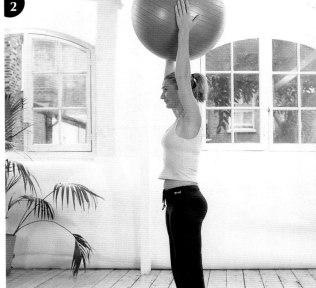

HOOVER

This is a really great exercise for improving upper-body strength. You will also be working the abdominals hard to maintain your neutral spine position.

> **THE AIM:**
> To tone and strengthen your upper-body muscles.

❶ Start over the ball on your hands and knees. Walk yourself out on your hands until the ball is underneath your thighs.

Once there, maintaining neutral spine position, lower yourself on to your elbows and link your fingers so that your forearms form a triangle. Engage your abdominal contraction and make sure that your body is in a straight diagonal line from your shoulders to your toes.

❷ Keeping the diagonal line straight, slowly roll yourself forwards so that you are lowering your nose over your hands towards the floor in front of you. Slowly roll yourself back to your starting position. Repeat 8–10 times.

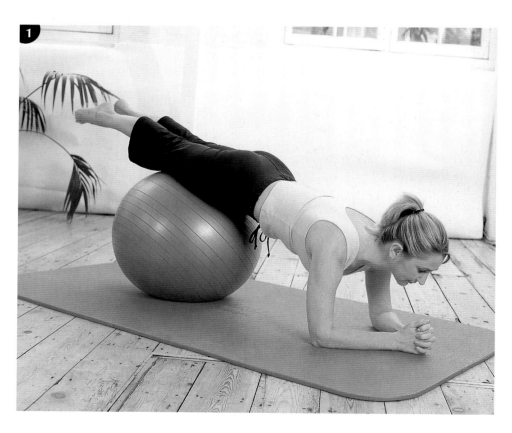

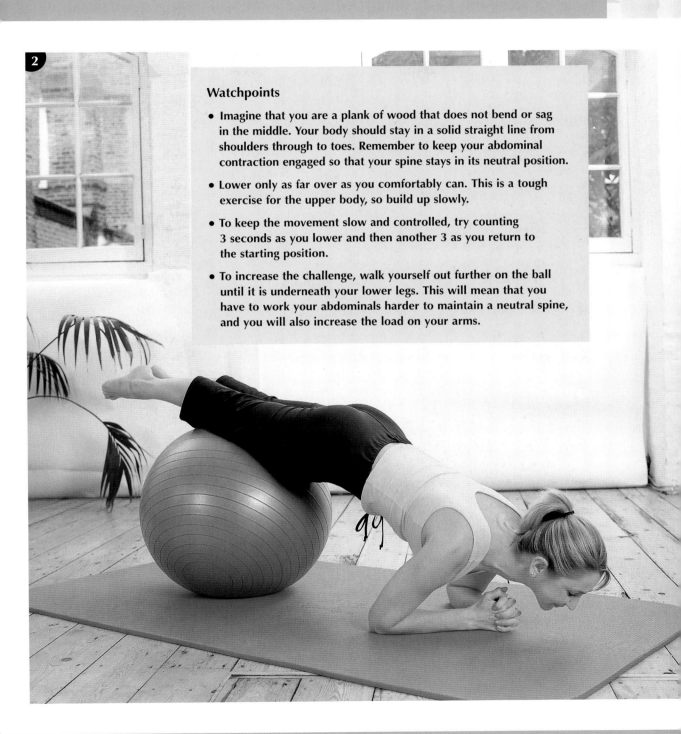

2

Watchpoints

- Imagine that you are a plank of wood that does not bend or sag in the middle. Your body should stay in a solid straight line from shoulders through to toes. Remember to keep your abdominal contraction engaged so that your spine stays in its neutral position.

- Lower only as far over as you comfortably can. This is a tough exercise for the upper body, so build up slowly.

- To keep the movement slow and controlled, try counting 3 seconds as you lower and then another 3 as you return to the starting position.

- To increase the challenge, walk yourself out further on the ball until it is underneath your lower legs. This will mean that you have to work your abdominals harder to maintain a neutral spine, and you will also increase the load on your arms.

TRICEPS DIPS

THE AIM:
To tone and strengthen the backs of your arms.

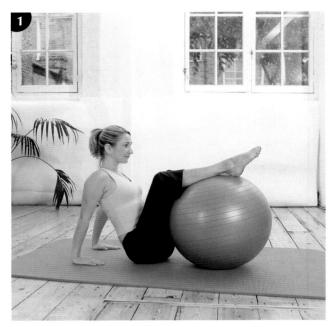

❶ Start seated on the floor with your feet up on the ball. Walk the ball in so that it is close to your bottom. Place your hands on the floor behind you with your fingers pointing in towards your bottom.

❷ Take your weight on to your arms. Bend your elbows, keeping your back straight, and then straighten your arms as you come back to the starting position. Repeat 10–15 times.

TO PROGRESS:

❸ *Progression 1* Repeat step 1. Once in position lift your bottom slightly off the floor by taking your weight on to your arms. Keeping your bottom lifted, bend your elbows as before, and then straighten back to the starting position. Repeat 10 –12 times.

❹ *Progression 2* Start seated on the front edge of the ball with your feet hip-distance apart. Place your hands on the centre of the ball behind you, with your fingers pointing in towards your bottom. Lift your bottom slightly off the ball.

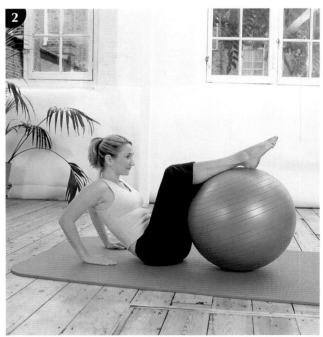

❺ Bend your elbows, lowering your bottom down the front of the ball, then straighten your arms again, returning to your starting position. This exercise is much more challenging with your hands on the ball as you are having to stabilise yourself with your arms at the same time. Repeat 8–10 times.

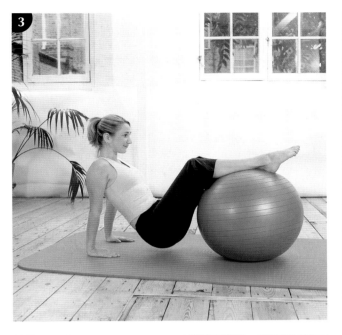

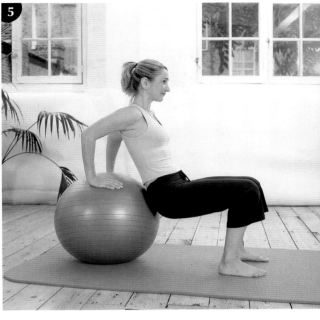

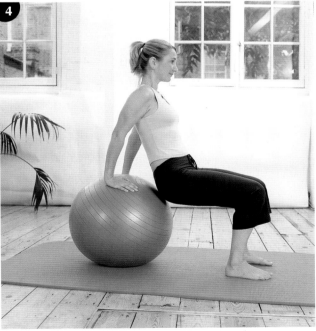

Watchpoints

- If you try the progressions, make sure that you bend and straighten your elbows rather than lowering your whole body from the shoulders.

- If your bottom is on the floor, make sure that you take your weight back on to your arms as they bend.

- If you take the dip with your hands on the ball, make sure that you stabilise yourself before you begin and keep the movement small at first until you feel more confident.

- Breathe out on the effort, in this case as you straighten your arms.

CHEST PRESSES

THE AIM:
To tone and strengthen the muscles in your chest and the backs of your arms, using the ball as a bench and light weights for resistance.

❶ Start seated on the ball, holding your weights. Slowly walk your feet out, allowing the ball to roll up your spine until it is underneath your shoulder blades and is supporting your head and neck. Your hips should be level with your knees. Engage your abdominal contraction to keep your spine in neutral. Hold the weights just above your shoulders.

❷ Extend your arms directly up towards the ceiling, keeping your shoulder blades pushed into the ball. Bend your arms back to their starting position and repeat 10–15 times. Then lower the weights in to your chest and walk yourself up to a seated position.

Watchpoints

- **Do not lock your elbows.**

- **Remember to keep your abdominal contraction engaged so that your spine stays fixed in its neutral position.**

- **Make sure that your head and neck are totally supported by the ball. Do not let your head hang over the back of the ball.**

- **Keep your shoulder blades in contact with the ball throughout.**

- **Keep the weights in line with your chest; do not allow them to move around as you extend your arms.**

- **Make sure that your hips stay lifted throughout; do not allow them to sag.**

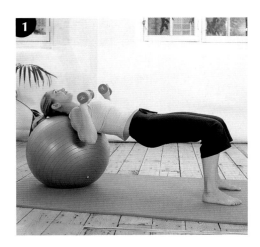
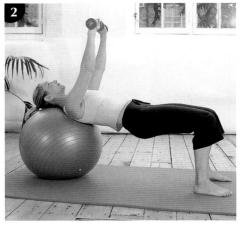

FLIES

THE AIM:
To tone and define your chest and shoulders, using the ball as a bench and light weights for resistance.

1 Start seated on the ball, holding your weights. Slowly walk your feet out, allowing the ball to roll up your spine. Keep walking until the ball is underneath your shoulder blades, supporting your head and neck. Your hips should be level with your knees. Hold the weights in front of your chest, with your arms extended and palms facing each other. Engage your abdominal contraction to keep your spine in its neutral position.

2 Keeping your arms straight (but elbows slightly relaxed), open them out to the sides. Now slowly return them to their starting position. Repeat 10–15 times.

Watchpoints

- **Keep your elbows slightly relaxed throughout.**

- **Make sure that your head and neck are completely supported by the ball.**

- **Do not let the weights move around; keep them directly in line with your chest.**

- **Remember to keep your abdominal contraction engaged so that your spine stays fixed in its neutral position.**

- **Your hips should stay lifted, and your knees should be directly over your ankles.**

- **Keep the movement slow and controlled at all times.**

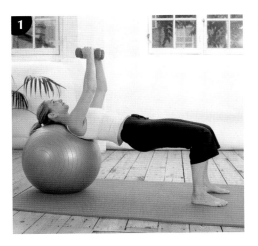

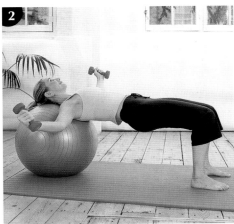

REVERSE FLIES

THE AIM:
To tone and strengthen your rear shoulder muscles, using the ball as a bench and light weights for resistance.

1 Start on your hands and knees over the ball. Pick your weights up off the floor and hold them in line with your nose, with your palms facing each other. Make sure that your elbows are slightly bent so that your arms are rounded.

2 Open your arms out to the side as wide as you can without lifting your chest. Keep your elbows rounded. Lower your arms back to the starting position. Repeat 10–15 times.

Watchpoints

- Keep your abdominal contraction engaged so that your spine stays fixed in its neutral position, preventing movement in the torso.

- Keep your focus down to the floor so that your neck stays in line with the rest of your spine.

- Keep your arms rounded to prevent you from taking too much of the weight into the elbow joint.

- Try not to hold your breath. Breathe out as you lift the arms and in as you lower.

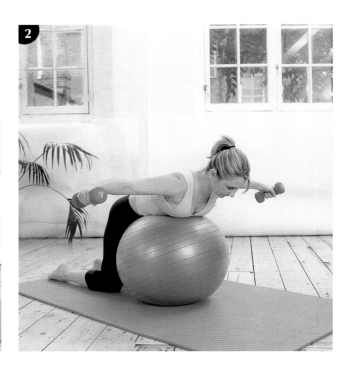

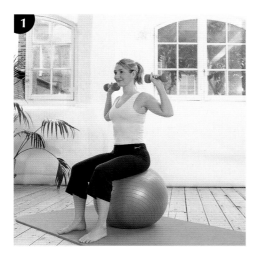
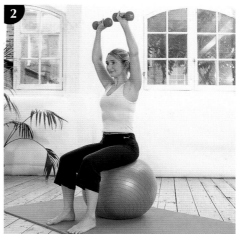

SEATED SHOULDER PRESSES

THE AIM:
To tone and strengthen your shoulders
and the backs of your arms, using the
ball as a bench and light weights for
resistance.

❶ Start seated on the centre of the ball
with your feet hip-width apart and your
knees over your ankles. Make sure that
your spine is in neutral position and that
your abdominal contraction is engaged.
Hold your weights so that they are just
above your shoulders, with your elbows
out to the sides.

❷ Push the weights up so that they almost
touch together above your head. Make sure
that the weights stay in front of the centre
line of your body. Bend your elbows,
bringing your arms back to their starting
position. Repeat 10–15 times.

Watchpoints

- Make sure that you are sitting in
  the centre of the ball, right up on
  your sitting bones.

- It is especially important here to
  remember to keep your abdominal
  contraction engaged so that your
  spine stays fixed in its neutral
  position whilst you are lifting the
  weights above your head.

- Try not to let your arms swing
  around. They should go directly up
  and down, straight into position.

- Your weights are too heavy if you
  find that you have to start moving
  your torso to lift them. Find a
  weight that you can lift with
  control and precision.

- Breathe out as you push your arms
  up and in on the way down.

SEATED SIDE RAISES

THE AIM:
To tone and strengthen your shoulder muscles, using the ball as a bench and light weights for resistance.

❶ Start seated on the centre of the ball with your feet hip-width apart and your knees over your ankles. Make sure that your spine is in neutral position and your abdominal contraction is engaged. Hold your weights with your arms down by your sides and your elbows slightly relaxed.

❷ Raise your arms to shoulder height, keeping them extended but still with your elbows slightly relaxed. Slowly lower them back to your sides. Repeat 10–15 times.

Watchpoints

- Make sure that you are seated in the centre of the ball, right up on your sitting bones.

- Be careful not to allow your torso to swing backwards and forwards when lifting and lowering your arms; keeping your abdominal contraction engaged will ensure that your spine stays fixed in its neutral position, helping you to avoid this.

- Make sure that the movement is slow and controlled. It will not be as effective if you throw your arms up and down and allow momentum to take over.

- Breathe out as you lift your arms and in as you lower.

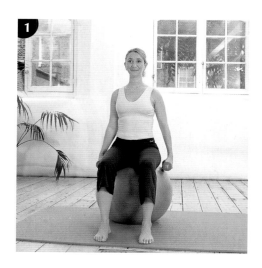

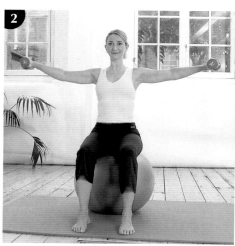

PEC DECS

THE AIM:
To tone and open out your chest muscles, using the ball as a bench and light weights for resistance.

1 Start seated on the centre of the ball with your feet hip-width apart and your knees over your ankles. Make sure that your spine is in neutral position and your abdominal contraction is engaged. Holding your weights, lift your bent arms up in front of you, elbows level with your shoulders, palms facing each other.

2 Keeping your arms bent at right angles, open them out to the sides. Your elbows should still be level with your shoulders and your palms now facing forwards. Close your arms together again, keeping your elbows lifted. Repeat 10–15 times.

Watchpoints

- Make sure that you are seated in the centre of the ball, right up on your sitting bones.

- Keep your arms bent at right angles throughout.

- Think about squeezing the muscles in the chest as you close your arms in front.

- Keep your abdominal contraction engaged so that your spine remains fixed in its neutral position.

- The movement should be slow and controlled throughout.

- Imagine that your shoulder blades are sliding down your back, keeping your shoulders pushed down.

- Do not allow your torso to move as your arms open and close.

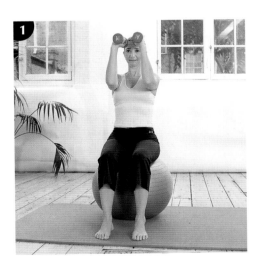

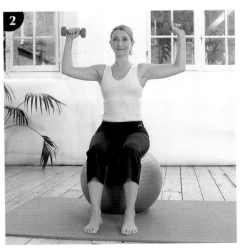

TRICEPS EXTENSIONS

THE AIM:
To tone and define the backs of your arms, using the ball as a bench and light weights for resistance.

1 Start seated on the centre of the ball with your feet hip-width apart and your knees over your ankles. Make sure that your spine is in neutral position and your abdominal contraction is engaged. Holding a weight in your right hand, reach it as far down your back as you can. Use your left hand to push back the elbow while holding it in place.

2 Extend your right arm, keeping your elbow pushed back level with your ear using your left hand. Bend your elbow again, returning to the starting position. Repeat 10–15 times on each side.

Watchpoints

- **Remember to keep your abdominal contraction engaged so that your spine stays fixed in its neutral position; it is tempting otherwise to arch your back as your arm goes overhead.**

- **Keep your elbow pushed back by your ear; use the opposite hand to hold it in place.**

- **When you extend your arm, try not to lock the elbow. This will help to avoid putting too much pressure on the joint.**

- **Keep the movement slow and controlled throughout.**

- **Breathe out as you extend your arm and in as you lower it.**

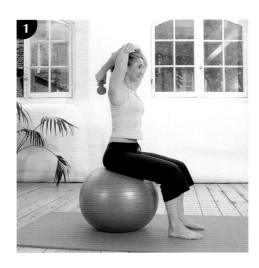

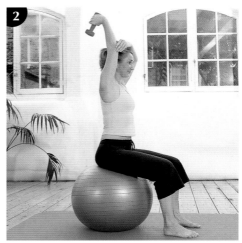

BICEPS CURLS

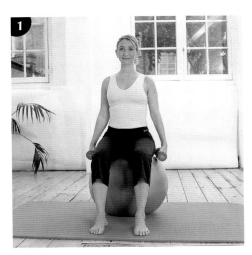

THE AIM:
To tone and strengthen your arms, using the ball as a bench and light weights for resistance.

❶ Start seated on the centre of the ball with your feet hip-width apart and your knees over your ankles. Make sure that your spine is in neutral position and your abdominal contraction is engaged. Hold one weight in each hand and start with your arms by your sides, palms facing in.

❷ Curl your hands up towards your shoulders, rotating your palms so that they are now facing your body. Slowly lower your hands back to their starting position. Repeat 10–15 times.

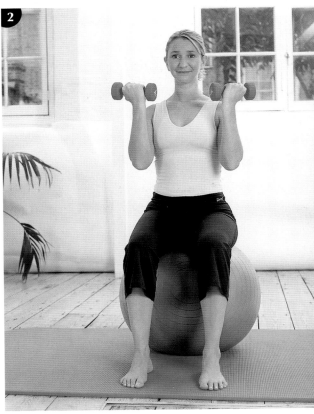

Watchpoints

- **Keep your torso still. Do not lean forwards and backwards as you lift and lower your arms.**

- **Keep the movement controlled throughout. Try not to swing your arms as this momentum will make the exercise less effective.**

- **Stay seated on the centre of the ball, right up on your sitting bones.**

- **Breathe out as you lift and in as you lower.**

CHAPTER 8: FULL-BODY INTEGRATION

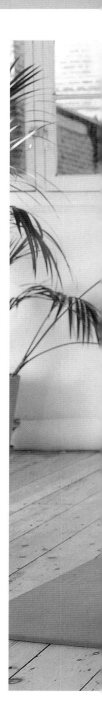

The exercises in this section challenge the body's ability to work as a whole integrated unit to achieve a 'full-body' focus and awareness where every single muscle plays its part. You will need to work your abdominals hard in order to stabilise your lower back and maintain a strong shoulder position to support your upper body and ensure good posture, whilst all the time co-ordinating other isolated movements of the limbs.

These exercises are great for building body awareness. When you begin to understand the physicality of your body through exercise, you soon reap the benefits in the other areas of your life. You will find that you are able to address the way that you sit when driving your car, or when you work at your PC, for example. And being aware of the way in which you hold yourself at social gatherings could actually make you look considerably taller, leaner and more confident.

Try to feel the role that each area of your body plays in maintaining the positions in these exercises. Do not concentrate only on the areas that are moving, but keep a check on the rest of your body: are you still lengthening, supporting, stabilising and pulling in? Enjoy learning how you can be in total control of your body and conscious of every movement that you make.

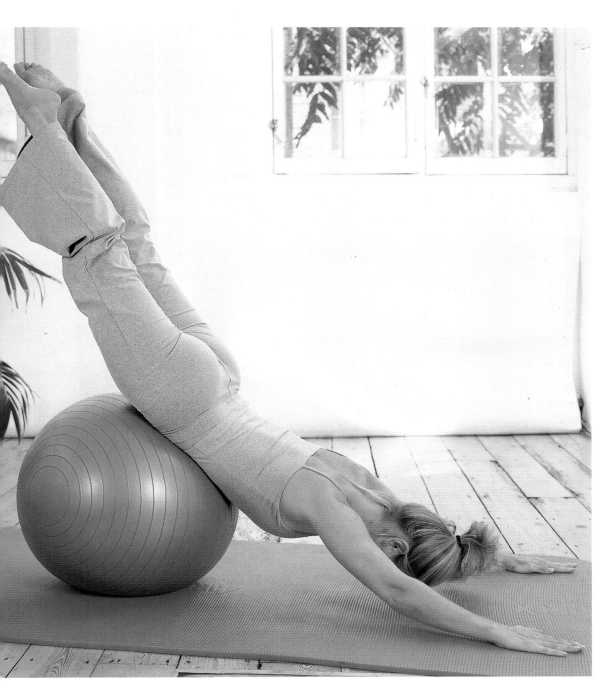

SWAN DIVES

This exercise feels fantastic when you get it right as it integrates the whole body.

❶ Start over the ball on your hands and knees. Walk yourself out forwards on to your hands. Keep walking, allowing the ball to roll down your legs. Stop when the ball is underneath your thighs, making sure that your hands are directly under your shoulders. Your abdominal contraction should be engaged to maintain a neutral spine position and prevent the lower back from sagging at any time.

❷ Keeping your arms extended, push the heels of your hands into the floor, allowing the ball to roll backwards until you are in a lengthened position from hands to toes. Keep your head and legs in line with the rest of your body. Push the heels of your hands into the floor again as you roll yourself forwards until the ball is back underneath your thighs and your hands are directly under your shoulders. Repeat 6–8 times. To come off the ball, slowly walk your hands back in until you are once again over it on your hands and knees.

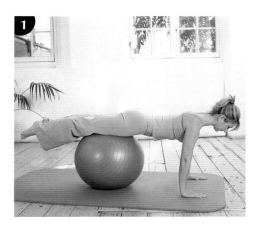

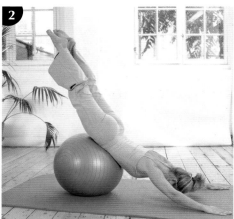

Watchpoints

- **Think long, rather than arching your lower back as you push away. Imagine that your hands and feet are being pulled in opposite directions.**

- **Breathe out as you push away and in as you return.**

- **If you find that your hands slip on the floor and you do not have a non-slip mat, try putting your hands on the floor in front of a wall. This does make the exercise a little easier, though, so keep it as a last resort!**

HEDGEHOG ROLLS

Stick with this one. Although it can be difficult at first, it feels great once you have mastered it!

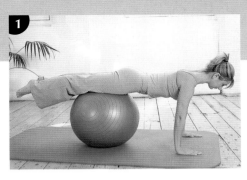

THE AIM:
To co-ordinate abdominal strength with upper-body strength, whilst maintaining stability through the body as a whole and challenging your balance skills.

1 Start over the ball on your hands and knees. Walk yourself out forwards on to your hands, allowing the ball to roll down your legs until it is underneath your thighs. Make sure that your hands are directly under your shoulders and your abdominal contraction is engaged. Keep your elbows slightly relaxed.

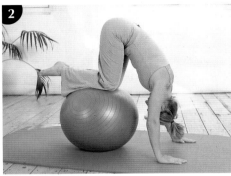

2 Keeping your shoulders directly over your wrists, bend your knees, lift your bottom up towards the ceiling and roll the ball in towards your chest. Focus on using your abdominals to initiate the movement. Slowly roll the ball out again, but only about three quarters of the way back to your starting position as this helps you to maintain the abdominal contraction and stops you from

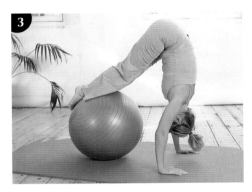

taking a rest between each repetition. Repeat 8–10 times. Then slowly walk yourself back down on to your hands and knees.

TO PROGRESS:

3 Repeat step 1, only this time keep your legs straight as you roll the ball in, pulling the body into a pike position. Lift your bottom high into the air. Keeping control throughout, lower three quarters of the way back to your starting position. Repeat 8–10 times.

Watchpoints

- **Maintain control throughout the movement, counting 4 seconds as you pull up and 4 as you lower.**

- **Keep your navel pulled in towards your spine throughout.**

- **Breathe out as you roll the ball in and in as you lower.**

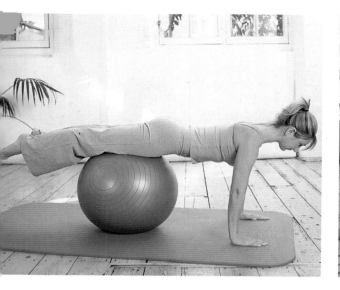

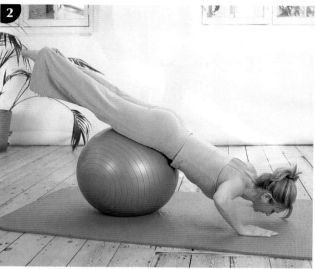

PRESS-UPS

This is much more challenging than the good old press-up on the floor!

Repeat 8–10 times. To come off the ball, walk your hands back in until you are again over the ball on your hands and knees.

THE AIM:
To tone your chest and triceps, whilst maintaining a neutral position and stabilisation throughout your body.

TO PROGRESS:

❶ Start over the ball on your hands and knees. Walk yourself out forwards on to your hands. Keep walking, allowing the ball to roll down your legs. Stop when the ball is underneath your thighs. Make sure that your hands are directly under your shoulders and your abdominal contraction is engaged to maintain a neutral spine position. Keep your elbows slightly relaxed.

❷ Bend your elbows, lowering your nose towards the floor. Extend your elbows again, pushing through the heels of your hands.

❸ Repeat step 1 as above, only this time continue walking out over the ball until it is underneath your lower legs. The further you walk out, the harder this exercise becomes. Make sure that you only walk out as far as you can whilst still maintaining a neutral position in your spine. Continue with step 2 as above.

● To progress still further, if you feel that you are keeping your spine neutral with the ball under your lower legs, you could try walking out even further until the ball is underneath the balls of your feet. This is very challenging, so try it only once you have built up enough strength to stabilise your body in this position.

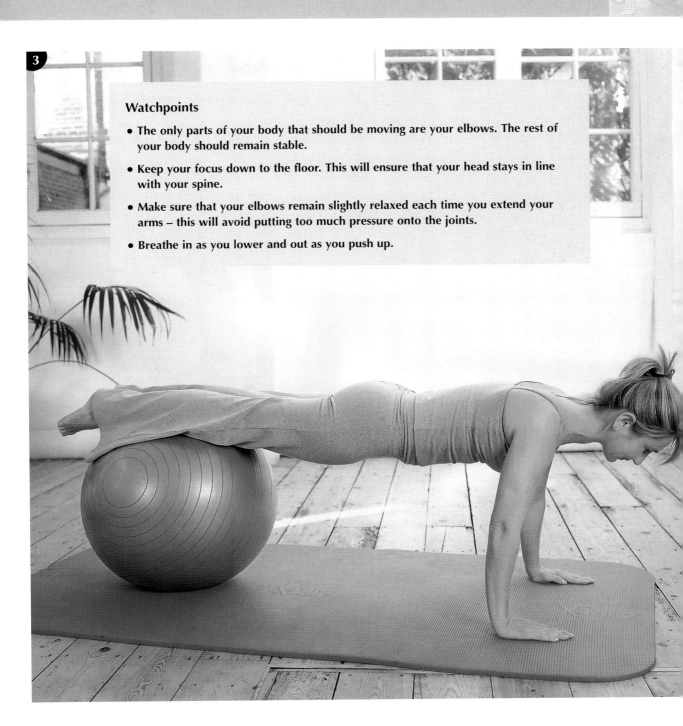

3

Watchpoints

- The only parts of your body that should be moving are your elbows. The rest of your body should remain stable.

- Keep your focus down to the floor. This will ensure that your head stays in line with your spine.

- Make sure that your elbows remain slightly relaxed each time you extend your arms – this will avoid putting too much pressure onto the joints.

- Breathe in as you lower and out as you push up.

KNEE BALANCE

You will be amazed at how quickly your balance improves if you do this on a regular basis…and don't worry about falling off – we all do it!

THE AIM:
To challenge your core balancing skills and stability muscles.

❶ Start over the ball on your hands and knees. Walk yourself out on to your hands, allowing the ball to roll down your legs and stopping when it is under your thighs. Engage your abdominal contraction.

❷ Bend your knees and roll the ball in, sitting yourself back on to your heels.

❸ If you feel comfortable with increasing the balance challenge, try to take your hands away from the floor and place them on the ball. Use them to help stabilise the ball.

❹ If you feel ready for more of a challenge, take your hands off the ball and lift yourself up on to your knees. Take your arms out to the sides to aid balance. Reverse the process to bring yourself off the ball.

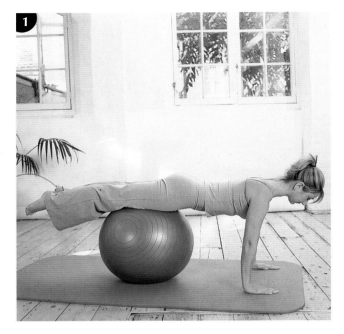

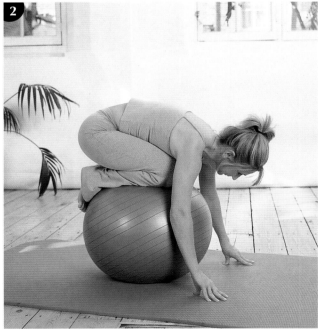

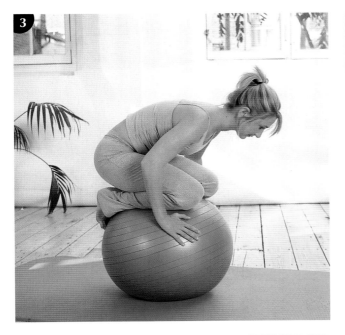

Watchpoints

- Take the balance only as far as you comfortably can. Make sure that you have cleared space around you so there is nothing to hurt yourself on if you roll off the ball. Until you feel more confident, you can always try this exercise holding on to something or someone.

- To gain a wider base of support on the ball make sure that your knees are at least hip-width apart.

- Keep your body strong; the more you turn to jelly, the less balance you will have.

- Focus on a fixed point at eye level. This will help you to remain balanced.

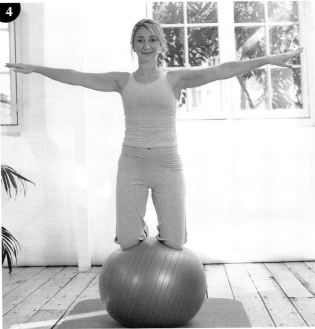

OPPOSITE ARM AND LEG RAISES

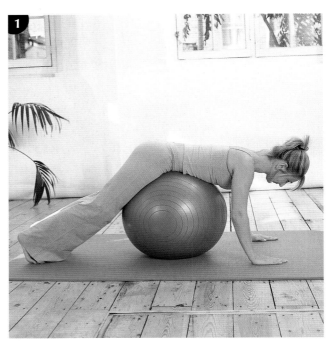

THE AIM:
To tone the muscles in your arms, torso and backs of the legs, and to integrate the whole body in practising core stability balance and neutral posture.

1 Start over the ball on your hands and knees. Walk yourself a little further forwards so that you are supported on your hips. Make sure that your weight is distributed evenly between your hands and feet.

2 Extend your right arm and left leg away from you along the floor. When you have lengthened as far as possible, allow them to lift away from the floor until they are parallel with it. Think of it as lengthening rather than lifting. Keep lengthening as you lower back to your starting position. Repeat with the left arm and right leg. Repeat 4–5 times on each side.

TO PROGRESS:

3 Repeat step 1 as above, then extend your right arm and both legs away from you until they are parallel with the floor in a balanced position. Slowly lower into your starting position, ready to repeat on the other side. Repeat 4–5 times on each side.

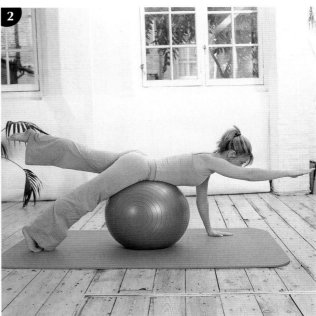

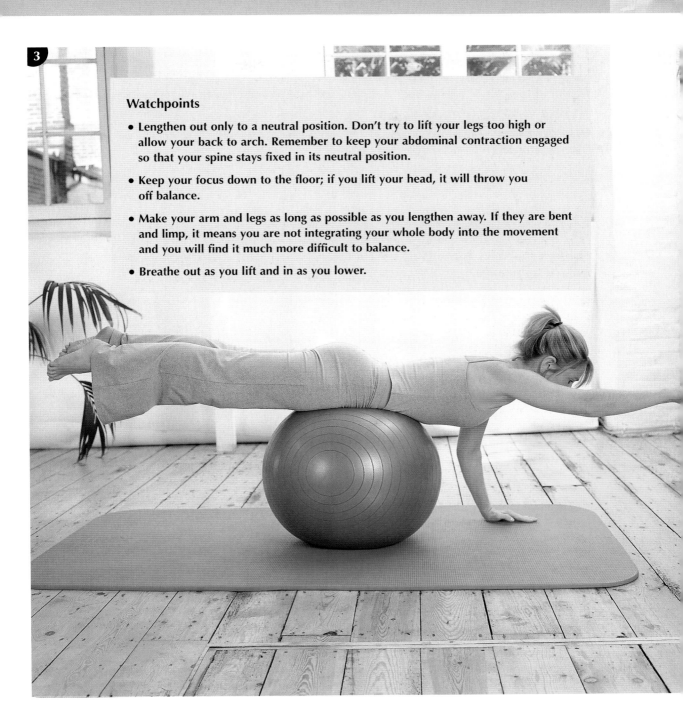

3

Watchpoints

- Lengthen out only to a neutral position. Don't try to lift your legs too high or allow your back to arch. Remember to keep your abdominal contraction engaged so that your spine stays fixed in its neutral position.

- Keep your focus down to the floor; if you lift your head, it will throw you off balance.

- Make your arm and legs as long as possible as you lengthen away. If they are bent and limp, it means you are not integrating your whole body into the movement and you will find it much more difficult to balance.

- Breathe out as you lift and in as you lower.

CHAPTER 9: STRETCH AND RELAX

We are all born with fantastic flexibility – think of how effortlessly a baby will put a foot in his or her mouth, for example. But the more we contract and strengthen our muscles, the more they shorten. Then, of course, there is the ongoing battle with the ageing process, in which the connective tissue actually becomes tighter. With stretching, however, you can help to maintain a good level of flexibility throughout life.

We all know how pleasing that first stretch of the morning is, so why is it that so many people either forget or just don't like to stretch after exercise? In its own way, stretching is as important as any other part of a workout, and it is essential to realise this. As well as improving your range of movement, it will also increase the oxygen content of your muscles, which, in turn, helps to flush out the lactic acid that is partly responsible for muscle soreness after exercise.

Of course, stretching does not only have to be done as part of a workout; it can also be done in isolation, on the days when you don't really feel like an exercise session. It can help to revamp a tired body or mind and is a great way to de-stress and relax. You can even get into the habit of doing gentle stretches with your ball as you watch television in the evening.

The ball makes some simple stretches even more effective. Working on the round surface gives you a much greater range of motion than on the floor. It is comfortable to work with and there is always the added balance challenge thrown in.

When you do the exercises in this section, try to make each stretch last at least as long as is specified, but longer if you feel comfortable doing so. Ease into position gently, starting cautiously until your muscles feel warm. When you are in the stretch try to take deep breaths and relax into it. The more you relax, the more you will feel your body naturally move deeper into the stretch. Do not bounce and go only as far as you comfortably can. If you notice that your muscles start to shake, this means that you have gone too far. Stretching really is a pleasure, and these exercises should help you to enjoy it.

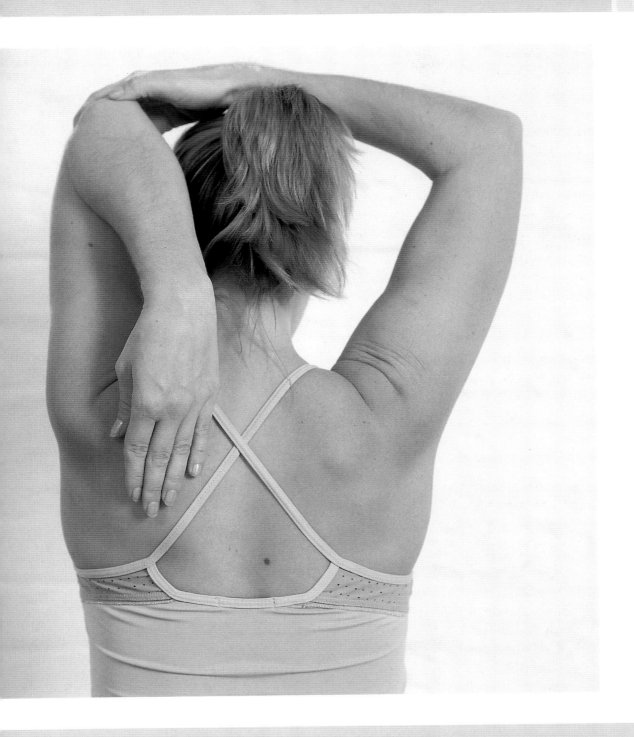

HAMSTRING STRETCH

The hamstrings are three muscles running down the back of each thigh. It is important to stretch them and to improve flexibility in this area as tight hamstrings can be a contributory cause of bad posture and lower-back pain. Ease yourself in gently if you are not used to stretching.

THE AIM:
To stretch and lengthen your hamstrings.

❶ Start on your back with both legs resting on the ball. Walk the ball in so that it is quite close to your bottom. Extend your right leg up towards the ceiling and, if you can, take hold of it with both hands. If you can't manage this, try using a towel or a dressing-gown belt to help you reach your lower leg. Gently ease the leg towards your body, keeping it extended but not locked. Hold for 30–50 seconds if you can. Relax your leg back down on to the ball. Repeat on the other side.

Watchpoints

- **Make sure that your tailbone remains on the floor at all times.**

- **Do not try to force the stretch. Just take it as far as is comfortable and try to relax into it. You will feel the stretch naturally increasing as the muscles relax.**

- **Avoid taking any tension into the upper body.**

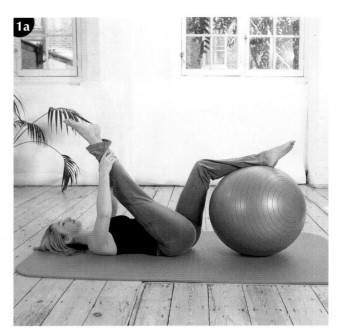

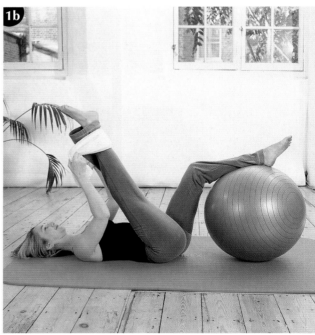

ALTERNATIVE HAMSTRING STRETCH

If you found the previous stretch difficult or uncomfortable, this version is an effective alternative.

THE AIM:
As before.

1 Start seated on the ball with your feet hip-width apart and your knees over your ankles. Place your hands on your thighs and make sure that your spine is in neutral position and your abdominal contraction is engaged. Extend your legs by pushing the ball backwards and tilt your body forwards so that you are leaning into the stretch. Try to keep your back lengthened. Hold for 20–30 seconds.

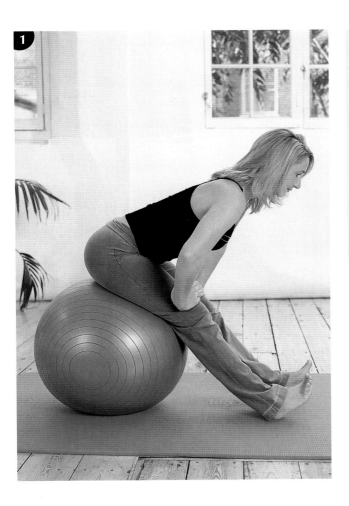

Watchpoints

- **Make sure that you don't lock your knees; keep them slightly relaxed.**

- **Visualise lengthening through the crown of your head (see page 16) so that your spine stays lengthened.**

- **Remember to keep your abdominal contraction engaged so that your spine stays fixed in its neutral position; this prevents arching in the lower back.**

FROG STRETCH

This is a great stretch where you don't have to put in any effort – just let gravity take its course!

1 Start on your back with the soles of your feet together and resting on the ball. Keep your arms relaxed and slightly away from your body. Allow your knees to open out gently to the sides. Relax and take deep breaths, allowing gravity to ease open your inner thighs. As you feel your muscles relax, try easing your feet towards your groin area a tiny bit at a time. This will increase the stretch. Stay in the stretch for at least 30–50 seconds, and if you feel comfortable you can relax in this position for as long as you want to.

> **THE AIM:**
> To stretch your inner-thigh muscles.

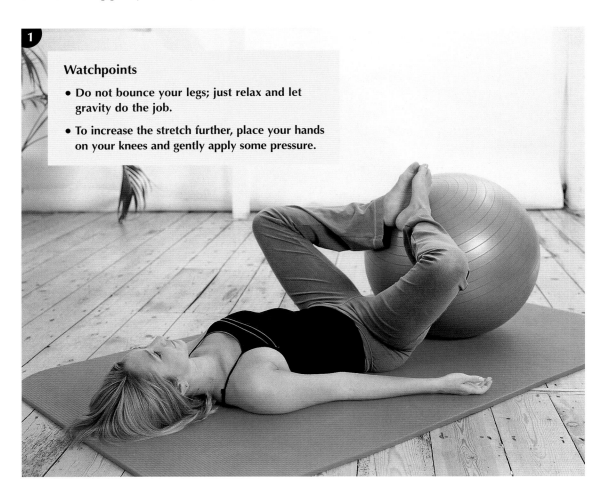

1

Watchpoints

- **Do not bounce your legs; just relax and let gravity do the job.**

- **To increase the stretch further, place your hands on your knees and gently apply some pressure.**

HIP STRETCH

In this exercise the ball controls the intensity of the stretch. Its great doing it this way as it avoids taking tension into the upper body as you would with the traditional version of this exercise, pulling your legs in with your hands.

THE AIM:
To stretch your hip rotators and your bottom.

❶ Start on your back with both legs resting up on the ball. Cross your right ankle over your left thigh, keeping the knee open. Use your left foot to roll the ball in towards your bottom until you feel a stretch deep in your right hip and buttock. Hold for at least 30 seconds, then roll the ball out slightly to release the tension. Repeat on the other side.

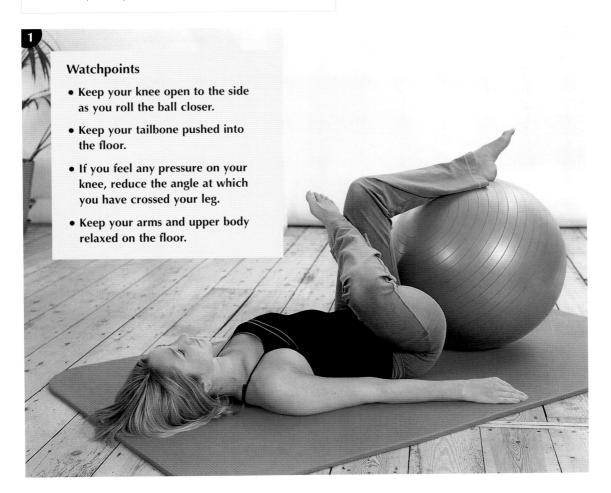

1

Watchpoints

- **Keep your knee open to the side as you roll the ball closer.**

- **Keep your tailbone pushed into the floor.**

- **If you feel any pressure on your knee, reduce the angle at which you have crossed your leg.**

- **Keep your arms and upper body relaxed on the floor.**

SIDE STRETCH

Only with the round surface of the ball is it possible to achieve this supported side stretch where you can almost wrap yourself around the ball.

THE AIM:
To stretch the whole side of your body.

---

❶ Start in a kneeling position with the ball on your right side and extend your left leg out to the side. With the ball as close to the side of your body as possible, reach your right arm over it, resting it on the floor on the other side. Lengthen your left arm over your head, reaching over your right side into a side bend. Hold the stretch for 30–50 seconds or longer if you feel comfortable. Return to your kneeling position and repeat on the other side.

Watchpoints

- Try to relax your body over the ball rather than taking all of your weight into your supporting knee.

- Keep your hips and shoulders square to the front.

- Take the stretch only as far as you comfortably can and be especially careful if you suffer with back problems.

- Try not to take any tension into your neck. If necessary, you can support your head with your right hand (or your left when you are repeating on the other side).

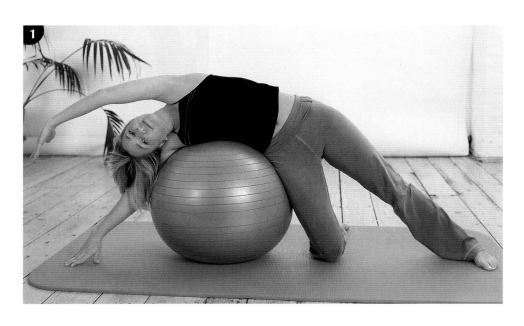

SIDE STRETCH WITH CHEST LIFT

This is a great stretch for releasing any tension in the upper back and chest areas. After you have done it you will feel as though these areas have been magically opened up.

THE AIM:
To stretch your sides, chest and upper back.

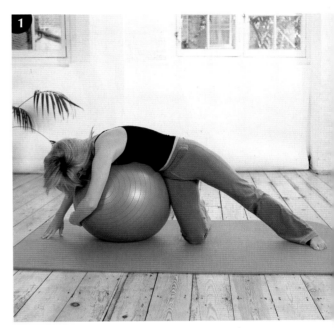

❶ Start in a kneeling position with the ball on your right side and extend your left leg out to the side. With the ball as close to the side of your body as possible, reach your right arm over it, resting it on the floor, and lengthen your left arm over your head, reaching over your right side into a side bend. Drop your chest and face on to the ball and hug it with your left arm. Hold for 15–20 seconds.

❷ Open your left arm back to its side bend position and then open it even further by taking it slightly behind your body until you feel a stretch down the left side of your chest. Hold for 15–20 seconds. Repeat each position 2–3 times, then repeat on the other side.

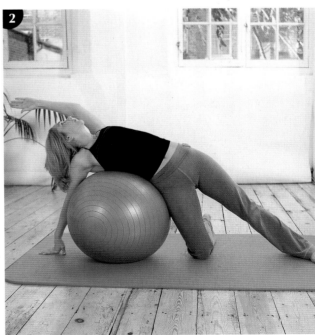

Watchpoints

- **Take deep breaths, relaxing into each position.**

- **Reach as far as is comfortable, especially on the back stretch.**

- **Relax your weight into the ball to avoid placing too much pressure on your supporting knee.**

- **Keep your abdominal contraction engaged so that your spine stays fixed in its neutral position.**

SPINAL TWIST

This is a lovely relaxing stretch. You will feel all the tension slip away from around your spine and hip area.

THE AIM:
To stretch your hip and outer-thigh muscles and to release the tension from the muscles around your spine.

❶ Start on your back with both heels resting up on the ball. Make sure that your knees are together and aligned over your hips. Extend your arms out to the sides at shoulder height with your palms facing down.

❷ Slowly allow your knees to lower towards the right side, making sure that you keep both shoulder blades pushed into the floor. Slowly bring your knees back to the centre, then repeat on the other side. Repeat 2–3 times on each side.

Watchpoints

- **Move slowly into this stretch, keeping control of the movement at all times.**

- **If your knees reach as far as the floor, you can relax in the position for 10–15 seconds before returning to the centre.**

- **Your shoulders must stay pushed into the floor, with your chest facing the ceiling.**

- **Remember to keep your abdominal contraction engaged so that your spine stays fixed in its neutral position.**

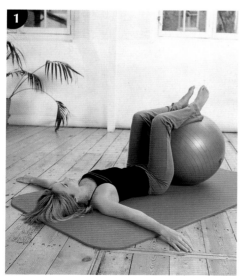
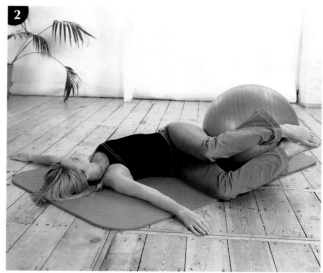

HIP FLEXOR STRETCH

A great stretch for hip flexibility. Use the ball to take some of your weight until you feel more comfortable with this one.

> **THE AIM:**
> To stretch your hip flexor muscles.

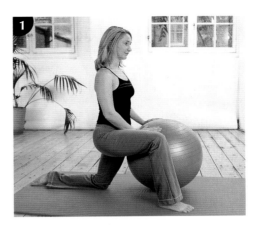

❶ Start in a kneeling position with the ball in front of your legs. Bring your right leg forwards, placing your foot flat on the floor so that your knee is bent up in a right angle. Rest your hands on the ball.

❷ Roll the ball out slightly, taking your weight forwards into your left hip. Use your hands on the ball to steady yourself. Hold the stretch for 20–30 seconds, then repeat on the other side.

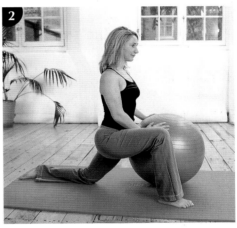

TO PROGRESS:

❸ Repeat step 1. Whilst steadying yourself as in step 2, curl the toes of your left foot under and extend your left leg, so the you rest on the ball of the foot in a lunge position. Hold for 20–30 seconds, then lower back on to your knee and change to the other side.

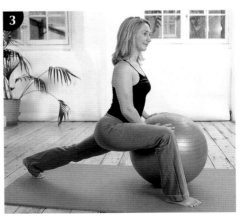

Watchpoints

- **Make sure that your supporting knee always stays vertically aligned with your ankle.**

- **Keep your torso upright; do not allow your body to collapse over the ball.**

- **If your knee is on the floor, try to avoid placing too much weight directly on the joint.**

INNER-THIGH STRETCH

Ease into this stretch very carefully and go only as far as you comfortably can. Do not worry how wide apart your legs are – you will be amazed at how quickly your flexibility will improve.

THE AIM:
To stretch your inner-thigh muscles.

❶ Start seated on the floor with your legs open as far as is comfortable and the ball placed in between them. Rest your hands lightly on the ball and sit up tall.

❷ With your hands, gradually roll the ball away from your body until you feel a stretch up your inner thighs. You may also feel it in your lower back. Hold the position for 10–15 seconds. If you feel that you can progress, roll the ball out a little further and hold the stretch for another 10 seconds. Slowly roll the ball all the way back in and relax your legs.

Watchpoints

- **Only take your legs out as far as your flexibility will comfortably allow.**

- **As you walk your hands out, make sure that your knees stay facing the ceiling. Do not allow them to roll forwards.**

- **Once in the stretch, try to relax your torso and take long, deep breaths.**

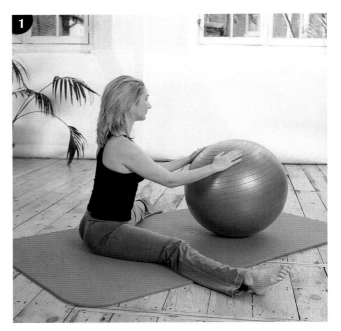

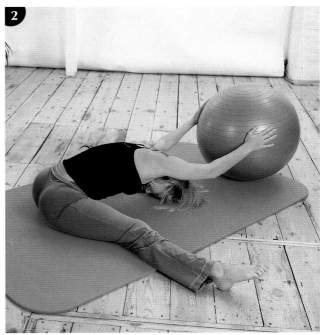

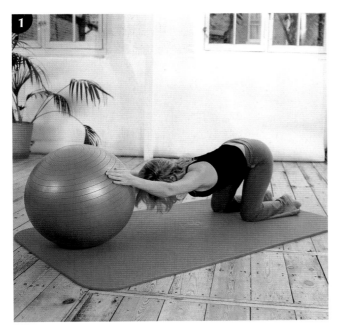

THREAD THE NEEDLE

This stretch is widely used in yoga to relieve tension in the upper body. It is called thread the needle in reference to the arm action as it passes underneath the body.

THE AIM:
To stretch the muscles in your shoulders and back.

1 Start in a kneeling position in front of the ball. Place your hands on top of the ball and roll it out until your hips are over your knees and your bottom, shoulders and head are all in a straight line.

2 With your left hand on top of the ball, thread your right arm under your left so that it reaches away from your body. Keep actively reaching as you hold this position for 10–15 seconds or as long as you comfortably can. Place your right hand back on to the ball and repeat on the other side.

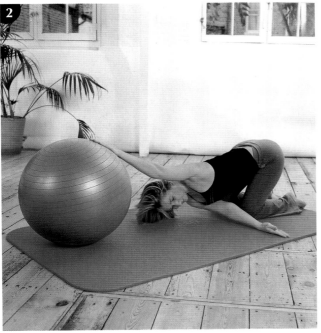

Watchpoints

- Make sure that your hips are aligned over your knees.

- Take your focus down to the floor so that your head stays in line with your spine.

- As you hold the stretch, keep the feeling of reaching away from your body with your arm.

THIGH STRETCH

This is excellent for stretching the fronts of your thighs, easing away that tired-leg feeling. It is a must if your workout included any squats.

> **THE AIM:**
> To stretch the muscles in the fronts of your thighs.

❶ Start over the ball on your hands and knees. Walk your hands out slightly, taking your knees off the floor so that the weight is evenly distributed between your hands and feet.

❷ Bring your right heel towards your bottom and take hold of the foot with your right hand. Keep both hips in contact with the ball. Push your hips into the ball to increase the stretch. Hold for 10–15 seconds or longer if you wish. Relax your leg back down. Repeat on the other side.

Watchpoints

- **Try not to strain your upper body to reach your foot. If it's a struggle, try using a towel or dressing-gown belt to help you to reach and hold on to your foot.**

- **Keep your hips and shoulders square to the floor.**

- **Focus down to the floor to keep your neck in line with the rest of your spine.**

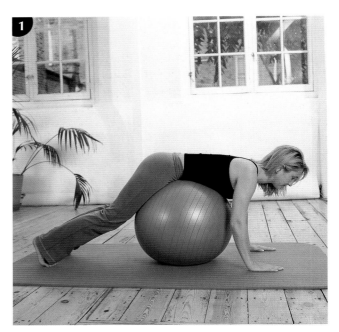

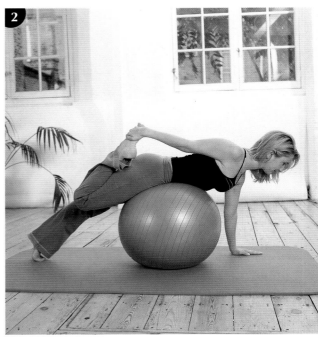

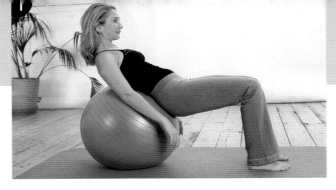

CHEST/FULL-BODY STRETCH

This is a most pleasurable stretch as you release all tension through the whole body.

❶ Start seated on the ball with your feet hip-width apart and your knees over your ankles. Walk your feet forwards, allowing the ball to roll up your spine. Stop when the ball is underneath your lower back.

❷ Bend your knees and drop your hips towards the floor. Rest your head on the ball.

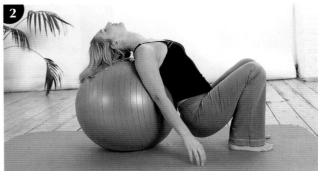

❸ Roll backwards on the ball until your chest is facing the ceiling. Open your arms out to the sides. You will feel a stretch across the chest here. Hold for 15–20 seconds. You will need to stabilise yourself on the ball.

❹ From this position reach your arms overhead and extend your legs as far as you comfortably can. Hold for 15–20 seconds. To come out of the stretch, bring your arms down to your sides, bend your knees, dropping your hips to the floor, then lift your head off and walk back up to your seated position.

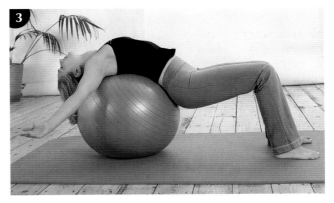

Note: if you suffer with back problems, do not attempt the full-body stretch.

Watchpoints

- **Roll only as far back into the stretch as you comfortably can.**

- **As you come out of the stretch don't try to lift your head off the ball before you have bent your knees all the way back down. You may strain your neck by attempting to do so.**

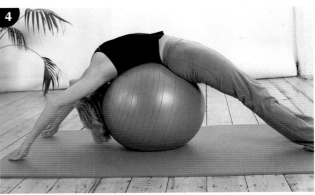

TRICEPS STRETCH

This stretch relaxes the backs of your arms and is especially worth doing after completing the upper-body strength section, which works the triceps particularly hard.

THE AIM:
To stretch the triceps muscles in the backs of the arms.

1 Start seated on the ball with your feet hip-width apart, your knees over your ankles and your spine in neutral position. Engage your abdominal contraction. Reach your right hand down your back as far as you can and gently push back on the elbow with your left hand. Hold the stretch for 10–15 seconds. Release your arm and repeat on the other side.

Watchpoints

- **Try not to allow your back to arch as you reach down it.**

- **Push back on your arm only as far as you comfortably can.**

- **If you are flexible in the shoulders, instead of pushing back on your elbow you could try to reach your other hand up your back and link the fingers together instead.**

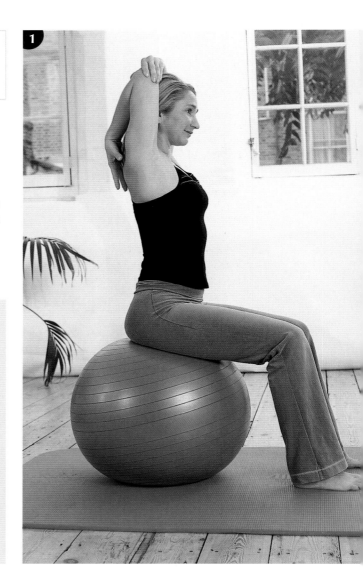

Relaxation

At the end of a hard workout you need to relax. Let's face it, you deserve it and it is highly beneficial to take some time to let go of any tension before you continue your other activities. Relaxing with the ball is very comforting, so even on days when you don't complete a workout you may enjoy the positions that follow, just to give you a little 'time out'. Letting go is very difficult at first and you may find it impossible to stop thoughts from constantly running around your mind. But as in any other exercise, with practice you will improve.

RELAXATION POSITION 1

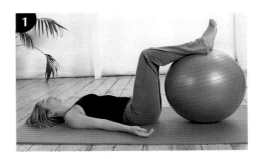

❶ Lie on your back with your feet resting up on the ball and your knees bent. Relax your arms by your sides. Close your eyes.

❷ Draw gentle circles with the ball before rolling it out so that your legs are extended. Allow your whole body to relax. Breathe in through your nose and out through your mouth. Imagine that your breath is gold in colour and picture its journey into your lungs, nourishing your whole body and then out through your mouth. Try to visualise this cycle until your whole body has absorbed the golden breath and it reaches out to your fingertips and down to your toes. Stay relaxed here for as long as you like. Now start slowly waking up your body, bringing awareness to each part. Start with your toes by giving them a wiggle, work up to your ankles and then to the calf muscles, tensing them slightly, then allowing them to relax again. Continue to work up your body until you reach the crown of your head. When you are ready, slowly open your eyes and sit up in your own time.

RELAXATION POSITION 2

This position is good if you find it uncomfortable to lie on your back. It is almost a foetal position and gives you the same sense of wellbeing.

❶ Start kneeling in front of the ball, then drape your body over it, relaxing your head and neck. Allow your body to wrap around the ball, moulding to its shape. Continue as with step 2 in relaxation position 1, above, then slowly bring yourself off the ball.

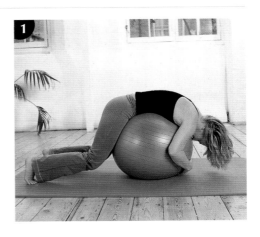

CHAPTER 10: ALL ABOUT EATING

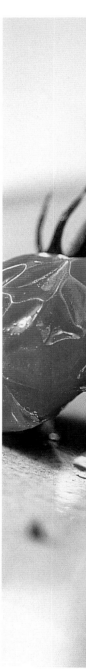

Although complicated by the many faddy diets we see advertised these days, the concept of weight loss should not be a difficult one: if you consume more calories than you expend, you will gain weight; if you expend more calories `than you consume, you will lose weight. It really is that simple.

Personally, I love my food. In fact at a lunch meeting regarding this book my editor even said to me, 'Wow, it's so refreshing to see a fitness expert who actually eats!' Food is a huge part of everyone's life, but what so many people forget are the actual reasons for eating. Food and water are our fuel: they provide our bodies with the nutrients that we need to function efficiently. Some foods have a lot more to offer than others, but ultimately each of the main food groups should be represented in a balanced diet.

One of the most positive steps you can take in trying to achieve your weight-loss goal is to analyse and address the emotional triggers that drive you to open that fridge door when you're not even hungry. If you can change the negative habits, it will help you to choose foods that not only assist in weight loss, but also fight disease, make your skin look fresh and glowing and give you long-lasting energy.

This does not mean that you have to give up all of the foods that you enjoy. It is the combinations and quantities in which you eat them that matter. Foods that you need less of, for example, are those with a high sugar and fat content as they have very little nutritional value. So if you balance your diet, eating more of what your body needs and less of what it does not, you will naturally eat less fat and less sugar and your body weight will decrease as a result.

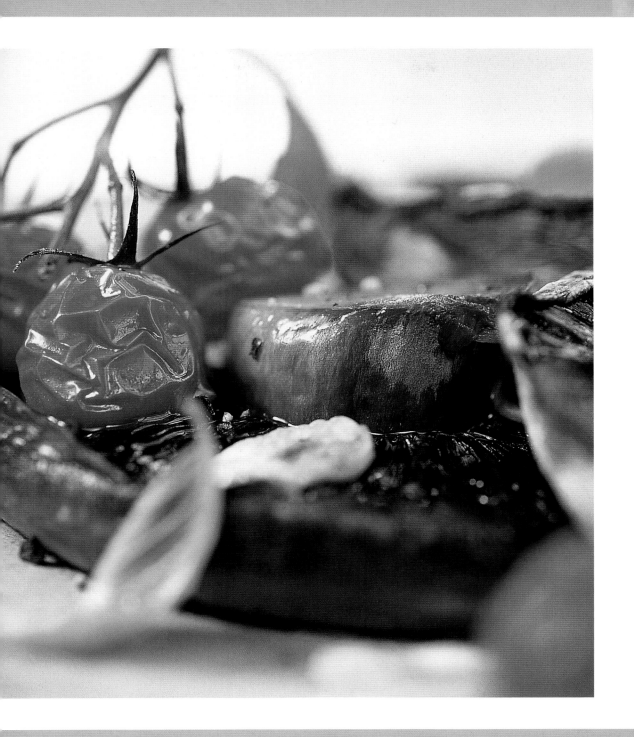

What is a balanced diet?

Starchy foods

This group includes bread, potatoes, cereals and grains. They are the core of a balanced diet, providing us with complex carbohydrates, fibre, vitamins and minerals. Choose the unrefined types (for example, wholemeal rather than white bread) and those that have little added fat and sugar.

Fruit and vegetables

Health guidelines suggest that we should try to eat at least five servings of fruit and vegetables per day (this does not include potatoes or sweet potatoes as these fall into the starchy foods category) and fresh or frozen are best. Small amounts of fruit juice or dried fruit can contribute to the five servings, but make sure that you choose the unsweetened varieties.

Meat, fish and protein alternatives

This group includes meat, fish, eggs, pulses, shellfish, nuts and seeds. Choose lean cuts of meat wherever possible and eat red meat in moderation. Always cut off any visible fat. Try to eat fish at least twice a week (one serving of which should be oily fish). Nuts seeds or pulses should also be included in your diet, particularly if you are a vegetarian.

Dairy foods

Dairy foods include milk, cheese, butter, cream and yoghurt. Eat foods from this group in moderation and always go for low-fat alternatives. Good choices are semi-skimmed or skimmed milk, cottage cheese, fromage frais and Greek-style yoghurts.

Sugary and high-fat foods

This group includes medium- and high-fat cheeses (that is, any that are not labelled 'half-fat' or 'reduced-fat'), cooking oils and fats, biscuits, cakes, crisps, pastries, sweets and other sweetened foods. Eat from this group sparingly as, apart from foods such as cheeses and sunflower oils, which are valuable in small amounts, these foods are of very little nutritional value. Eating less from this group and replacing it with food from other groups with less calorific value (such as fruit and vegetables) is a great way to start losing some weight.

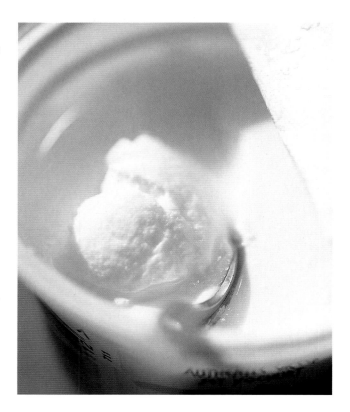

How do you go about choosing low-fat foods?

Doing the supermarket shopping is a stressful task in itself, and one that is made even more so by advertising and marketing. How do you pick your way through all the products whose labelling claims that they are 'low-fat', 'reduced-fat', 'lighter' or 'lite', to find those that are genuine?

Making a commitment to buying low-fat foods means reading the labels carefully. Be aware that of all the claims listed above, 'low-fat' is the only legally defined term: if a product is 'low-fat', it must contain less than 5g (1/5oz) fat per 100g (31/2oz) serving (with the exception of fat spreads which do not have to meet this guideline). Look for the information that matters – often printed as small as possible – and allow yourself enough time to compare and contrast products. Look at nutritional content and try to choose foods where the saturated fat is a small percentage of the total fat content.

Easy ways to cut down the fat in your diet

- Eat less of or cut out completely fats such as butter, margarine and hard fats.

- Choose extra-lean cuts of meat and trim off all the visible fat.

- Replace rich salad dressings, such as mayonnaise, salad cream and French dressing, with fat-free vinaigrettes.

- Eat less fried chips, sautéed or roasted potatoes and instead try baked or boiled potatoes, or replace potatoes with rice, couscous or pasta.

- Cook with spray oil or no fat at all. Use non-stick pans and where possible grill, bake or steam foods.

- Always roast or grill meat on a rack so that the fat can 'escape'.

Here is a sample label of a low-fat product. Note the total fat and saturated fat content.

Typical composition	Per 48g serving provides	100g provides
Energy	585kJ/138Kcal	1218kJ/287Kcal
Protein	3.9g	8.2g
Carbohydrate	27.7g	57.8g
of which sugars	9.1g	19.0g
Fat	1.2g	2.6g
of which saturates	0.5g	1.1g
Fibre	2.5g	5.2g
Sodium	0.2g	0.3g

Analyse what you eat

Before you can set about making changes to your eating habits, you need to take a closer look at where you are now. Start a food diary (see page 140) to help you keep track of everything that passes your lips for a whole week; remember to include things like sugar in tea and whether you use semi-skimmed instead of full-fat milk. You will find a section for snacks that don't fit into any of the meal categories, a section for drinks and also a section for emotions. This will help you to draw connections between how you feel and how you eat: it is not unusual, for example, to eat more when you are feeling particularly bored, or perhaps to crave sweets when you are premenstrual. By identifying emotional triggers we can start to put changes in place.

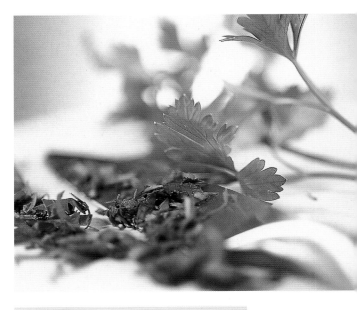

Where do you go from here?

You now know what a balanced diet contains. You know that to lose weight you need to cut down on high-fat and sugary foods. And you should also be aware how you you have gone wrong in the past. So now let's consider the way forward.

   On the following pages there are some recipes and a two-week meal planner to get you started on the right track. After two weeks you should find that your body is enjoying being fed wholesome nutritious foods, you will have discovered that low-fat foods can be just as enjoyable as the naughty alternatives, your blood-sugar levels should have regulated, which will mean fewer sweet cravings, and you will notice a difference in yourself both physically and mentally. You can then start to experiment with your own ideas, continue with the recipes here or maybe treat yourself to a low-fat cookbook for more inspiration – there are lots of good ones to choose from.

Food Alert

Every time you find that you are craving a snack, talk yourself through this mental checklist:

- **Am I really hungry?**

- **How am I feeling?**

- **Why do I want to eat?**

- **How will I feel if I do eat this?**

- **Will I regret eating this?**

If, having asked yourself these questions, you feel all right about going ahead, then do so. This way, at least you will have consciously made the decision to eat, and are therefore taking responsibility for doing it.

Recipes

This section includes a variety of delicious low-fat recipes for you to try. I have attempted to include foods and flavours that will appeal to a variety of palates, but there are countless books and websites with more ideas and suggestions (see page 144), so there should be no shortage of inspiration and no excuse to give up! In fact, once your body has had a chance to adapt to its new regime, you will find that you actually start to crave 'good' foods over high-calorie or junk foods.

BREAKFASTS

Fruit cocktail

Serves 2

Finely grated zest and juice of 1 orange

1 pink grapefruit

1 papaya

1 kiwi fruit

1 banana

Fresh mint, to garnish

1. Mix together the zest and juice from the orange in a large bowl.

2. Prepare the remaining fruit, cutting it into even-sized pieces. Add to the bowl, stirring to coat completely with the orange juice and zest. Cover and refrigerate overnight, then serve for breakfast with fresh mint leaves.

> **FOOD FACTS**
> Citrus fruits are a good source of vitamin C and are likely to reduce the risk of some cancers.

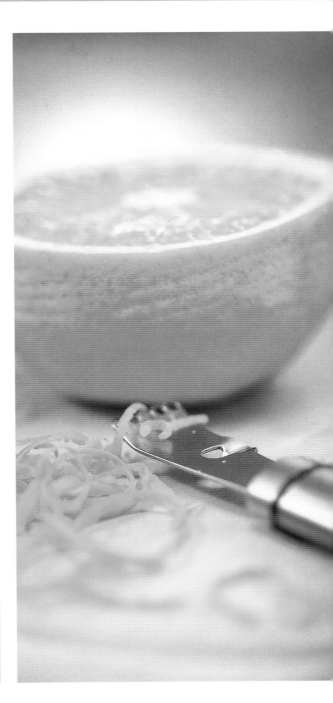

Red berry porridge

Serves 2

125g (4oz) berries (e.g. raspberries, blackberries)
500ml (17fl oz) water
1 tablespoon caster sugar
Pinch of salt
50g (2oz) semolina

1. Put a few berries to one side for a garnish, then purée the rest with the water using a blender or a hand-held mixer. Strain the mixture through a fine sieve into a saucepan.

2. Add the sugar and salt and place over a medium heat. Bring to the boil, then whisk in the semolina. Once the mixture is thoroughly blended, reduce the heat and leave to simmer for about 20 minutes, stirring frequently until it thickens.

3. Pour the porridge into bowls, leave to cool for 5 minutes, then garnish with the remaining berries.

Asparagus omelette

This delicious omelette is made with just the egg whites to keep it low in fat and cholesterol.

Serves 1

110g (3¾oz) trimmed asparagus
Salt and black pepper
4 medium egg whites
Handful of fresh parsley, chopped

1. Steam the asparagus for 8 minutes or until tender. Drain and season to taste.

2. Whisk the egg whites until they are frothy, but still pourable.

3. Heat the spray oil in a small frying pan. Pour in the egg whites and cook over a low heat until the bottom is firm.

4. Slide the omelette on to a plate, then place the asparagus in the pan and the omelette on top, uncooked side facing down. Cook for another few minutes until the bottom of the omelette has set and the asparagus is golden brown.

5. Serve asparagus side up.

Note: If asparagus is out of season, you could use spinach or broccoli instead.

FOOD FACTS
Asparagus is an extremely effective treatment for indigestion, and unlike drugs has no side effects.

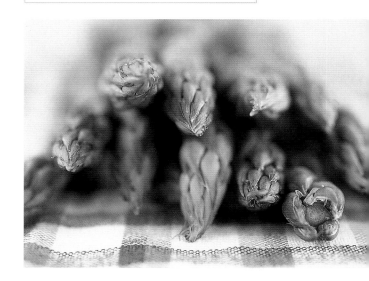

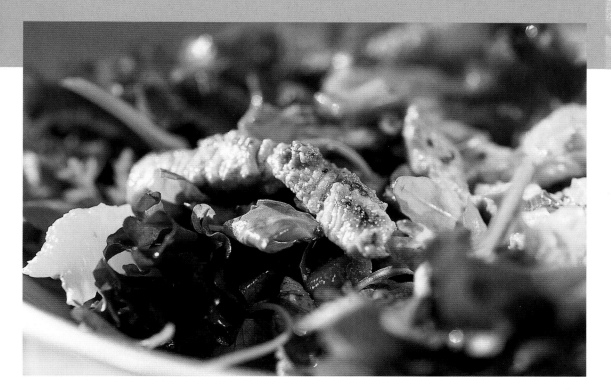

LUNCHES/STARTERS

Orange and turkey salad

This salad could also be served with a jacket potato for a main course.

Serves 4

FOR THE MARINADE:

2 large oranges

2 teaspoons honey

2 teaspoons wholegrain mustard

1 shallot, finely chopped

FOR THE SALAD:

500g (1lb) turkey breast, skinned

Spray olive oil, for cooking

Salt and black pepper

4 spring onions, sliced

125g (4oz) mixed salad leaves

1. To make the marinade, peel 1 of the oranges, removing all the pith. Divide into segments, cut the segments in half lengthwise and put them to one side. Squeeze the juice from the remaining orange into a bowl. Stir in the honey, mustard and shallot.

2. Cut the turkey breast into thin strips and add to the marinade, making sure that they are covered in the juice. Refrigerate for 15–20 minutes.

3. Heat a wok or non-stick pan, adding some spray oil. Stir-fry the turkey strips until they are cooked through and golden brown, adding the spring onions for the last few minutes. Season to taste with salt and black pepper. Pour in any remaining marinade and bring to the boil.

4. Divide the salad leaves between 4 plates and place the reserved orange segments on top. Spoon over the turkey mixture.

Spicy cottage cheese and tuna in a jacket

Serves 1

1 x 175g (6oz) baking potato

200g (7oz) tub of tuna and sweetcorn low-fat cottage cheese (buy it already mixed or mix your own)

1 spring onion, finely chopped

1/2 red pepper, deseeded and chopped

Dash of Tabasco sauce

Salt and black pepper

1. Preheat the oven to 200°C (400°F/gas mark 6) and bake the potato for 1 hour or until cooked. Alternatively, microwave for about 8–10 minutes, turning halfway through.

2. Mix together the cottage cheese, spring onion and red pepper. Add a dash of Tabasco sauce and season with salt and pepper.

3. Open the potato and top with the filling.

Spicy tomato and lentil soup

Serves 4

1 tablespoon olive oil

1 onion, finely chopped

1 garlic clove, crushed

1 teaspoon cumin seeds, crushed

2.5cm (1in) piece of fresh root ginger, finely chopped

500g (1lb) tomatoes, peeled and deseeded

125g (4oz) split red lentils

1 tablespoon tomato purée

1.2 litres (2 pints) vegetable stock

Salt and black pepper

1. Heat the olive oil in a large saucepan. Add the onion and cook until soft.

2. Stir in the garlic, cumin and ginger, followed by the tomatoes and lentils. Cook over a low heat for 4–5 minutes.

3. Stir in the tomato purée and the stock and bring to the boil. Lower the heat and allow to simmer for 30 minutes until the lentils are soft. Season with salt and pepper.

4. Pour the soup into a blender and purée. Return to a clean pan and reheat gently.

5. Serve in warmed bowls.

FOOD FACTS

Lentils and other pulses can substantially reduce blood cholesterol, high levels of which can increase the risk of heart disease.

Chestnut and mushroom terrine

This dish can also be served as a main course.

Serves up to 8

Spray olive oil, for cooking

175g (6oz) mushrooms, sliced

175g (6oz) red onions, thinly sliced

3 garlic cloves, finely chopped

8 whole chestnuts (unsweetened – canned or vacuum-packed)

1 egg, beaten

125g (4oz) wholemeal breadcrumbs

400g (14oz) chestnut purée (unsweetened – canned)

Grated zest of ½ orange

Juice of 1 orange

1 tablespoon chopped fresh parsley

1 tablespoon chopped fresh thyme

Salt and black pepper

Fresh coriander or basil, to garnish

1. Preheat the oven to 180°C (350°F/gas mark 4) and lightly grease a 1kg (2¼ lb) loaf tin.

2. Heat some spray oil in a large saucepan. Add the mushrooms, onions and garlic and fry over a medium heat for 7–8 minutes or until lightly browned.

3. Break the chestnuts into small pieces and stir them into the mixture, then add the egg, breadcrumbs, chestnut purée, orange zest and juice, parsley and thyme, using a wooden spoon to break up the chestnut purée. Add salt and pepper to taste and mix thoroughly.

4. Spoon the mixture into the prepared loaf tin, smooth over the top and bake for 45 minutes or until browned.

5. Leave to cool in the tin, then turn out on to a plate and cut into slices.

6. Garnish with the coriander or basil and serve with a mixed salad.

FOOD FACTS
Chestnuts have only a fraction of the fat content of other nuts and are still extremely tasty.

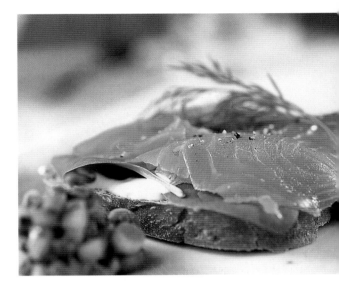

Open salmon and salsa sandwich

Serves 1

1 spring onion, chopped

5cm (2in) piece of cucumber, peeled deseeded and chopped

1 teaspoon chopped fresh dill

1 teaspoon capers, chopped

1 teaspoon French mustard

½ teaspoon caster sugar

Salt and black pepper

1 slice of fresh granary bread

1 teaspoon low-fat crème fraîche

Handful of baby spinach leaves

50g (2oz) smoked salmon slices

1. Mix together the spring onion, cucumber, dill, capers, mustard and sugar. Season with salt and black pepper.

2. Spread the bread with the crème fraîche,

arrange the spinach leaves on the bread and then place the salmon slices on top. Season well with black pepper.

3. Top the salmon with the cucumber and dill salsa and serve.

Mushrooms and cherry tomatoes

Serves 4

4 large, flat mushrooms

2 garlic cloves, finely sliced

Cherry tomatoes (about 4 or 5 per mushroom)

Spray olive oil, for cooking

Salt and black pepper

Fresh basil, to garnish

1. Preheat the oven to 220°C (425°F/gas mark 7).

2. Place the mushrooms on a lightly greased baking tray. Scatter the garlic over the mushrooms and arrange the tomatoes on top. Spray well with olive oil.

3. Season well with salt and black pepper, cover with foil and bake for 15 minutes.

4. Remove the foil and continue to bake for a further 15 minutes, until the vegetables begin to brown.

5. Garnish with basil leaves to serve.

> **FOOD FACTS**
> Tomatoes are rich in lycopene, a very powerful anti-cancer agent.

MAIN MEALS

Salmon and broccoli stir-fry on a bed of wholewheat noodles

Serves 2

200g (7oz) dried wholewheat noodles

Spray olive oil, for cooking

1 red pepper, deseeded and finely sliced

1 garlic clove, crushed

125g (4oz) broccoli florets

2 spring onions, sliced

2 x 125g (4oz) salmon fillets, skinned and cut into strips

1 teaspoon Thai fish sauce

2 teaspoons soy sauce

1. Bring a large saucepan of water to the boil and cook the noodles according to the instructions on the packet.

2. Using a large frying pan or wok, heat the oil and add the red pepper, garlic, broccoli and spring onions. Stir-fry over a high heat for 4 minutes.

3. Add the salmon, Thai fish sauce and soy sauce and cook for a further 4–5 minutes (or until the salmon is cooked through), stirring gently.

4. Drain the noodles and serve with the stir-fry.

> **FOOD FACTS**
> Wholewheat noodles contain complex carbohydrates. These are released slowly into the body, helping to keep your blood sugar and energy levels constant.

Spicy bean hotpot

Serves 4

225g (7^1/$_2$oz) button mushrooms

Spray olive oil, for cooking

2 onions, sliced

1 garlic clove, finely chopped

400g (14oz) can chopped tomatoes

1 tablespoon tomato purée

400g (14oz) can red kidney beans, drained and rinsed

400g (14oz) can haricot beans, drained and rinsed

100g (3^1/$_2$oz) raisins

1 tablespoon red wine vinegar

1 tablespoon Worcestershire sauce

1 tablespoon wholegrain mustard

1 tablespoon soft dark brown sugar

225ml (8fl oz) vegetable stock

1 bay leaf

Salt and black pepper

Fresh parsley, to garnish

1. Wash and slice the mushrooms. Put to one side.

2. Spray some oil into a large saucepan. Add the onions and garlic and cook over a gentle heat for 10 minutes or until soft.

3. Add all the remaining ingredients except the mushrooms, seasoning and parsley. Bring to the boil, then lower the heat and simmer for 10 minutes.

4. Add the mushrooms and simmer for another 5 minutes. Add salt and pepper to taste and serve sprinkled with the parsley.

Vegetable pasta

You can choose any combination of spring vegetables for this tasty dish.

Serves 4

250g (8oz) asparagus spears

125g (4oz) mangetout, trimmed

125g (4oz) baby corn

250g (8oz) baby carrots, trimmed

1 small red pepper, deseeded and chopped

250g (8oz) dried pasta shells

150ml (^{1}/$_4$ pint) low-fat cottage cheese

150ml (^{1}/$_4$ pint) low-fat yoghurt

1 tablespoon lemon juice

1 tablespoon chopped fresh parsley

Salt and black pepper

1. Steam or boil the asparagus, mangetout, baby corn, carrots and red pepper until tender. Drain.

2. Cook the pasta in a large pan of boiling water according to the instructions on the packet. Drain.

3. Put the cottage cheese, yoghurt, lemon juice and parsley into a blender, season with salt and pepper and process until smooth.

4. Put the creamy sauce into a large pan with the pasta and vegetables. Heat gently and stir thoroughly. Serve immediately.

Fish cakes with lemon sauce

These fish cakes are delicious served with a salad of tomatoes and sugar snap peas.

Serves 4

375g (13oz) potatoes, chopped

75ml (3fl oz) skimmed milk

Salt and black pepper

375g (13oz) salmon or haddock fillets, skinned

1 tablespoon lemon juice

1 tablespoon creamed horseradish

2 tablespoons chopped fresh parsley

Flour, for dusting

125g (4oz) fresh wholemeal breadcrumbs

Spray olive oil, for cooking

FOR THE SALAD:

Olive oil

Balsamic vinegar

1 teaspoon French mustard

Chopped fresh chives or 1 teaspoon dried Italian herbs

Handful of cherry tomatoes

Handful of sugar snap peas

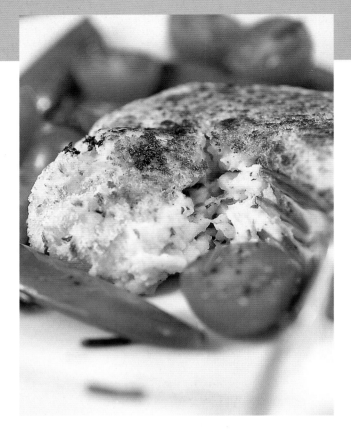

1. Cook the potatoes in boiling water until soft. Drain and mash, adding the milk. Season with salt and pepper to taste.

2 Purée the fish, lemon juice and horseradish in a blender. Mix in the potatoes and parsley.

3. With floured hands divide the mixture into 8 cakes and coat each one with the bread-crumbs. Chill in the fridge for 20 minutes.

4. Preheat the grill to medium and spray a little olive oil on to a clean grill pan to avoid sticking. Grill the fish cakes for about 5 minutes on each side, until golden brown.

5. To make the salad dressing, mix together the olive oil, balsamic vinegar, mustard and herbs and season to taste.

6. Chop the cherry tomatoes in half and arrange on a plate with the sugar snap peas. Drizzle over the salad dressing and then serve with the cooked fish cakes.

> **FOOD FACTS**
> The omega-3 fatty acids found in oily fish boast a whole range of health benefits: they reduce the likelihood of developing heart disease and blood clots and they also provide an anti-inflammatory action.

Beef and pepper stir-fry

Serves 4

250g (8oz) dried egg noodles

1 tablespoon sesame oil

325g (11oz) beef steak, cut into strips

500g (1lb) mixed peppers, deseeded and sliced

100g (3^1/$_2$oz) baby corn

200ml (7fl oz) beef stock

1 tablespoon soy sauce

2 slices of fresh root ginger, finely chopped

Pinch of Chinese five-spice

1 teaspoon cornflour

a handful of fresh coriander to garnish

1. Cook the noodles according to the instructions on the packet.

2. Heat the sesame oil in a wok and stir-fry the beef strips and peppers over a high heat until they are browned.

3. Add the baby corn and a little of the stock. Stir-fry for a further 2 minutes.

4. Add the soy sauce, ginger and five-spice. Add a little more of the stock and stir-fry for a further 2 minutes.

5. Add the cornflour to the remaining stock and add to the pan. Bring to a simmer, stirring continuously.

6. Sprinkle with coriander and then serve.

> **FOOD FACTS**
> Ginger is great for relieving indigestion and flatulence.

Moroccan lamb casserole

This dish is best served with couscous. A great warmer for those cold winter nights.

Serves 4

1 tablespoon olive oil

500g (1lb) lamb fillet, cubed

1 large onion, sliced

1 garlic clove, finely chopped

1 teaspoon ground cumin

1 teaspoon ground cinnamon

2 teaspoons flour

Salt and black pepper

1 sachet saffron strands

900ml (1^1/$_2$ pints) lamb stock

125g (4oz) dried apricots, chopped

50g (2oz) dried apple rings, chopped

400g (14oz) can chickpeas, drained and rinsed, or 250g (8oz) dried chickpeas, cooked

1 tablespoon lemon juice

1. Heat the oil in a wok. Add the lamb and cook on a high heat until browned. Remove and keep warm.

2. Stir-fry the onion for a few minutes until soft. Add the garlic, cumin and cinnamon and continue stir-frying for 1 minute.

3. Add the flour, stirring, then season with salt and pepper.

4. Return the lamb to the wok and add the saffron and stock. Stir, then add the dried apricots and apple rings, chickpeas and lemon juice.

5. Cover and simmer for 1 hour.

Potato, leek and tomato bake

Serves 4

750g (1½lb) potatoes, thinly sliced

2 leeks, sliced

3 large tomatoes, sliced

2–3 sprigs fresh rosemary, chopped

1 garlic clove, finely chopped

300ml (½ pint) vegetable stock

1. Preheat the oven to 180°C (350°F/gas mark 4) and grease a shallow ovenproof dish.

2. Place the potatoes in a pan of boiling water for 2 minutes. Drain well and layer them in the dish with the leeks and tomatoes, sprinkling some rosemary between each layer. End with a layer of potatoes.

3. Add the garlic to the stock and season with salt and black pepper. Pour the mixture over the potatoes, leeks and tomatoes.

4. Bake for 45 minutes or until the potatoes are soft and golden on top.

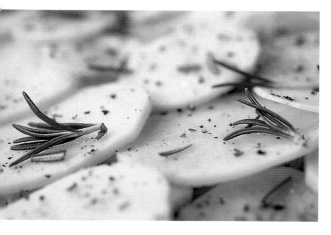

DESSERTS

Crunchy fruit layer

This is quick, easy and tasty – good enough to serve at a dinner party.

Serves 4

250g (8oz) raspberries (you can substitute any other fruit)

250g (8oz) low-fat natural yoghurt

75g (3oz) Swiss-style muesli

1. Keep 4 raspberries to one side for decoration, then divide the rest between 4 stemmed glasses.

2. Pour a spoonful of yoghurt into each glass.

3. Sprinkle a layer of muesli over the yoghurt, then repeat the layers, finishing with a layer of muesli.

4. Top each glass with a raspberry and serve within 20 minutes, or the muesli loses its crunch.

Eton mess

Serves 4

500g (1lb) strawberries

300g (10oz) low-fat Greek-style yoghurt

200g (7oz) tub low-fat strawberry fromage frais

4 meringue nests, broken into small pieces

1. Keep 4 strawberries to one side for decoration and chop the remainder.

2. Mix together the yoghurt and fromage

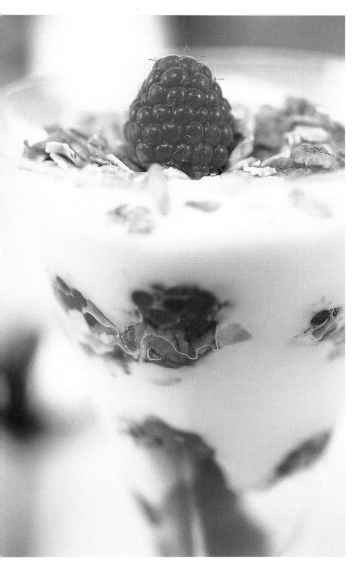

Poached pears in red wine

Serves 4

4 firm ripe pears
1 large glass red wine
2.5cm (1in) cinnamon stick
4 cloves
40g (1½oz) fruit sugar (fructose)

1. Peel the pears, cut them in half and remove the cores.

2. Put the pear halves in a saucepan with the wine, cinnamon, cloves and sugar. Spoon the wine over the pears, then add enough water just to cover them.

3. Cover the pan and simmer for 30 minutes or until the pears are tender.

4. Remove the pears from the pan with a slotted spoon and put them to one side, keeping them warm. Boil the remaining liquid until it has reduced and thickened. Remove the cinnamon and cloves.

5. Arrange the pears in 4 bowls and spoon the sauce over the top to serve.

frais, then gently fold in the broken meringue nests and the chopped strawberries.

3. Divide between 4 stemmed glasses and decorate each one with a whole strawberry. Chill for 15 minutes before serving.

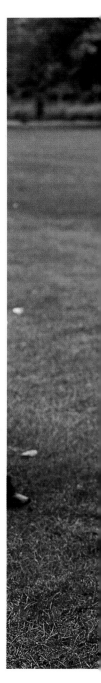

This chapter includes a two-week meal plan, a personalised food diary and also an exercise plan, so it's time to put it all together and get started on the new you. The first step is always the hardest, but once you incorporate these changes into your everyday life, they soon become second nature to you and will feel increasingly liberating.

Two-week meal plan

After you have used the food diary to analyse what you eat and where you are going wrong (see page 140), it is time to develop good habits. This two-week plan is based on a diet consisting of healthy, balanced, low-fat foods. Many of the recipes from the previous chapter are included, along with other simple dishes as suggestions. The idea is to initiate a change in your eating habits that, in tandem with your exercise ball programme, will help to bring about some fantastic results in both your body shape and your general well-being.

Exercise plan

To get you started I have put together a full-body toning programme, including the warm-up and stretch, to give you an idea of how to structure your workout. This does not include all of the exercises in the book, so once you have tried a few sample sessions, you can then go on to create your own programme, incorporating other exercises that you enjoy.

Remember that, whatever type of workout you choose, you must always stretch the muscles you have been working when you have finished. This will help you to prevent unnecessary injury.

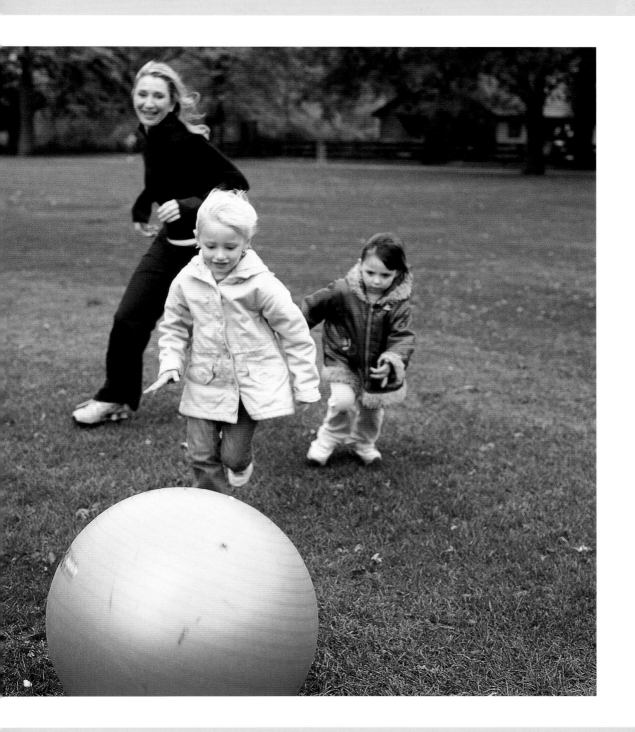

Two-week meal plan

Keep your portion sizes reasonable; serving your meals on a smaller plate will make it more difficult to pile it all on! Try to limit your alcohol intake to three or four units a week (one unit being equivalent to a small glass of wine) and avoid too much tea and coffee – one or two cups a day are enough, or try herbal teas instead. Stick to no-added-sugar squashes and fizzy drinks if you must drink them, and remember to drink lots of water. Use low-fat spreads and cheeses and either semi-skimmed or skimmed milk. If you feel that you need a snack between meals, try a piece of either fresh or dried fruit (but avoid those that are coated in honey or extra sugar), low-fat yoghurt, a raw carrot or a wholemeal cracker. And lastly, remember that if you are not sure what a food contains, always check the label.

WEEK 1

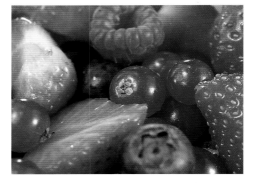

Monday
BREAKFAST
150g (5oz) tub low-fat natural bio yoghurt with a banana chopped in

LUNCH
Orange and turkey salad (page 125)

MAIN MEAL
Spicy bean hotpot (page 129)

Tuesday
BREAKFAST
50g (2oz) No-added-sugar muesli with semi-skimmed milk

LUNCH
80g (3¼oz) can of tuna in brine, drained, on a mixed leaf, tomato and cucumber salad with oil-free dressing

MAIN MEAL
Vegetable pasta (page 129)

Wednesday
BREAKFAST
Fruit cocktail (page 123)

LUNCH
Open salmon and salsa sandwich (page 127)

MAIN MEAL
Potato, leek and tomato bake (page 132)
1 slice of melon

Thursday
BREAKFAST
1 slice of wholemeal toast with low-fat spread and no-added-sugar jam.
1 orange.

LUNCH
Spicy cottage cheese and tuna in a jacket (page 126)

MAIN MEAL
Beef and pepper stir-fry (page 131)

Friday
BREAKFAST
Bran flakes with skimmed milk (or semi-skimmed, if preferred)

LUNCH
Mushrooms and cherry tomatoes (page 128)

MAIN MEAL
Grilled fish with new potatoes and broccoli

Saturday
BREAKFAST
150g (5oz) tub low-fat natural bio yoghurt with a banana chopped in

LUNCH
Large mixed salad with oil-free dressing, about 50g (2oz) low-fat cheese and a small granary roll

MAIN MEAL
Moroccan lamb casserole (page 131)

Sunday
BREAKFAST
Asparagus omelette (page 124)

Lunch
1 wholemeal pitta bread filled with mixed salad, oil-free dressing and 1 slice of cooked lean meat

Main meal
Roast beef with new potatoes, carrots and peas
Eton mess (page 132)

WEEK 2

Monday
BREAKFAST
Fruit cocktail (page 123)

LUNCH
Spicy tomato and lentil soup with 1 small granary roll (page 126)

MAIN MEAL
Salmon and broccoli stir-fry on a bed of wholewheat noodles (page 128)

Tuesday
BREAKFAST
No-added-sugar muesli with semi-skimmed milk

LUNCH
Spicy cottage cheese and tuna in a jacket (page 126), or try another low-fat jacket potato filling of your choice

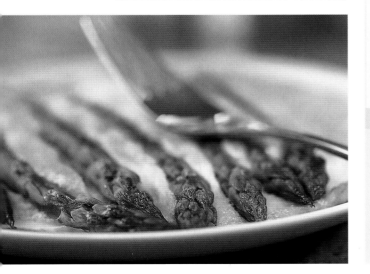

MAIN MEAL
Low-fat chicken curry (ready-made low-fat sauces can be found in all good supermarkets; use skinless chicken breast fillets and serve on a bed of rice
Crunchy fruit layer (page 132)

Wednesday
BREAKFAST
1 slice of wholemeal toast with low-fat spread and honey and 1 piece of fruit

LUNCH
Orange and turkey salad (page 125)

MAIN MEAL
Vegetable pasta (page 129)

Thursday
BREAKFAST
150g (5oz) low-fat tub natural bio yoghurt with a banana chopped in

LUNCH
1 wholemeal pitta bread, filled with mixed salad, oil-free dressing and 1 slice of cooked lean meat

MAIN MEAL
Potato, leek and tomato bake (page 132)

Friday
BREAKFAST
Red berry porridge (page 124)

LUNCH
Baked beans on 1 slice of wholemeal toast

MAIN MEAL
Fish cakes with lemon sauce (page 130)

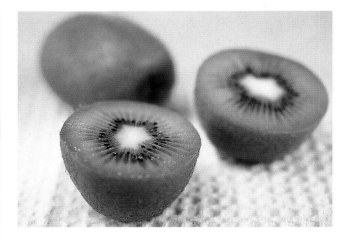

Saturday
BREAKFAST
Fruit cocktail (page 123)

LUNCH
Mushrooms and cherry tomatoes (page 128)

MAIN MEAL
Grilled fish with a jacket potato and green beans

Sunday
BREAKFAST
1 medium egg, poached on 1 slice of wholemeal toast with low-fat spread

LUNCH
1 slice chestnut and mushroom terrine (page 126) with 2 wholemeal crackers

MAIN MEAL
Roast chicken with new potatoes, spinach and butternut squash
Poached pears in red wine (page 133)

Your exercise regime

I recommend that you should aim for three sessions per week of aerobics with the ball (see page 22), as well at least two toning sessions. These should comprise toning exercises from each chapter, working each area of the body in turn. You may choose to work for longer on a particular area one day and then another the next; this is fine so long as you do not end up neglecting any one area. Stick with the basic levels for each exercise or try the progressions if you feel that you need more of a challenge – whatever works best for you.

It is also important to vary your workout; there are enough exercises in this book to make that possible and sometimes the exercises you find hardest are the ones that are doing you the most good, so keep that in mind when you are tempted to skip over the exercises you don't like! The set exercise plan on the following page will get you started...

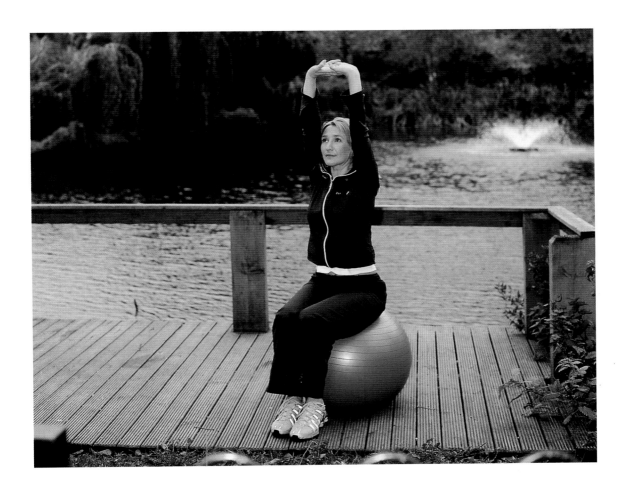

Exercise plan

WARM-UP

Foot taps	page 25
Half stand-ups	page 24
Jacks	page 26
Pendulum swings	page 30
Double arm circles	page 34
with double side step	

Note: You should do each of the above warm-up exercises for at least one minute.

THE EXERCISES

Squats against the wall	page 54
Spine twists	page 71
Trunk curls	page 38
Bottom squeezes	page 58
Trunk curls with knee lifts	page 42
Side-lying oblique lifts	page 44
Side-lying leg lifts	page 62
Back extensions	page 68
Press-ups	page 96

Hedgehog rolls	page 95
Hoover	page 80
Seated shoulder presses	page 87
Flies	page 85
Biceps curls	page 91
Triceps dips	page 82
Inner-thigh squeezes	page 59
Double leg lifts	page 63
Hamstring curls	page 64
Hip extensions	page 74
Reverse curls	page 47

STRETCH

Hamstring stretch	page 104
Hip stretch	page 107
Frog stretch	page 106
Side stretch	page 108
Triceps stretch	page 116
Chest/full-body stretch	page 115
Relaxation position 1	page 117

Food Diary

	Breakfast	Mid-am	Lunch	Mid-pm	Dinner	Drinks	Snacks	Emotions
Mon								
Tues								
Wed								
Thurs								
Fri								
Sat								
Sun								

Top tips to keep you going

- 15 sit-ups on the ball are equivalent to 100 on the floor, and will take you less than a minute.

- Get plenty of sleep. Lack of essential sleep will increase your levels of the stress hormone cortisol, which, in turn, stimulates appetite. Research has also found that we are more likely to store fats and sugars when we are tired.

- Eat off a blue plate – according to colour therapists, blue depresses the body's systems including, of course, your appetite.

- Trade in your sofa and try sitting on your ball instead whilst you watch television. Without even realising it you will be working muscles just to keep yourself from collapsing into a heap on the floor.

- Eat slowly. It takes 20 minutes for your brain to register that you are full, so if you savour your food, you may find that you can't even clear your plate.

- The more you do your toning exercises on the ball, the more you will increase the muscle mass in your body. This doesn't mean you will grow big, bulky muscles, but it does mean that your metabolism will work faster.

- Eat more spicy foods. We tend to eat these more slowly, so that often it takes less food to make us feel full. Spicy foods will also speed up your metabolism a little, so that you will burn more calories without lifting a finger.

- Zest it up! Cooking low-fat foods does not mean that you have to compromise on flavour. Stock up on herbs, spices, mustards and chutneys, and don't be afraid to experiment.

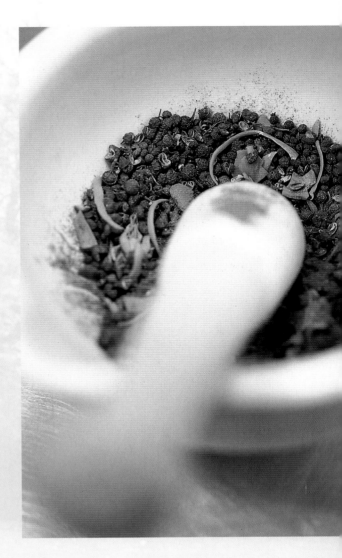

INDEX

RESOURCES

Ball Dynamics International
www.fitball.com
International suppliers of the ball

British Nutrition Foundation
www.nutrition.org.uk
Advice on nutrition

Fat Free
www.fatfree.com
Vegetarian low-fat recipe archive

Halfords
www.halfords.com
They sell a great electric pump that
plugs into your car lighter and blows
the ball up in no time at all

Health Canada
www.hc.sc.gc.ca/english/lifestyles
Canadian website including information on
staying both mentally and physically healthy

Healthy Living
www.healthyliving.gov.uk
Scottish website with information on healthy
eating, physical activity including case studies

IMC Vision
www.imcvision.com
On this website you can purchase any of
my Gymball or Pilates videos/DVDs. There
is also an extensive range of other good
quality, healthy-living programmes

Know Your Body Best
www.knowyourbodybest.com
800-881-1681
Canadian distributor of exercise balls and
other exercise equipment

Little Guru
www.littleguru.co.uk
Online lifestyle magazine

Living and Raw Foods
www.living.foods.com
A site that gives great information on
vegetarian foods and recipes

Low-Fat Recipes
www.low-fat-recipes.com
Lots of free low-fat recipes, nutrition advice
and cookbooks

Proactive Health
www.proactive-health.co.uk
Ball-related exercise equipment

The Physical Company
www.physicalcompany.co.uk
01494 769222
Balls, pumps, ball carry straps, mats and
other exercise equipment

The Soil Association
www.soilassociation.org
Bristol House
40-56 Victoria Street
Bristol BS1 6BY
A directory of outlets supplying organic
produce

USA Pro
www.usapro.co.uk
0116 2838181
Workout clothing and interesting lifestyle
facts on their website

www.fitballs.co.uk
Everything to do with the ball